Helping Elderly Relatives

Jill Eckersley is a freelance writer with many years' experience of writing on health topics. She is a regular contributor to women's and general-interest magazines, including *Women's Running, Women's Fitness, Slimming World* and other titles. *Coping with Childhood Asthma, Coping with Childhood Allergies, Helping Children Cope with Anxiety, Every Woman's Guide to Heart Health, Living with Eczema, Every Woman's Guide to Digestive Health, Coping When Your Child Has Cerebral Palsy, Coping with Snoring and Sleep Apnoea* and *Coping with Early-onset Dementia,* nine books written by Jill for Sheldon Press, were all published between 2003 and 2010. She lives beside the Regent's Canal in north London with her cat.

Overcoming Common Problems Series

Selected titles

A full list of titles is available from Sheldon Press,
36 Causton Street, London SW1P 4ST and on our website at
www.sheldonpress.co.uk

Overcoming Common Problems Series

Overcoming Common Problems Series

Overcoming Common Problems

Helping Elderly Relatives

JILL ECKERSLEY

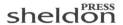
sheldon PRESS

First published in Great Britain in 2013

Sheldon Press
36 Causton Street
London SW1P 4ST
www.sheldonpress.co.uk

The author and publisher have made every effort to ensure that the external
website and email addresses included in this book are correct and up to date at the
time of going to press. The author and publisher are not responsible for the content,
quality or continuing accessibility of the sites.

British Library Cataloguing-in-Publication Data
A catalogue record for this book is available from the British Library

ISBN 978–1–84709–262–5
eBook ISBN 978–1–84709–263–2

Typeset by Caroline Waldron, Wirral, Cheshire
First printed in Great Britain by Ashford Colour Press
Subsequently digitally reprinted in Great Britain

Produced on paper from sustainable forests

To Mum and Dad,
Jeff and Mary Beavers of Southport,
who have always made wise decisions

Contents

Acknowledgements

I would not have been able to write this book without the help of the many people who shared both their professional expertise and personal experiences with me. I would especially like to thank Dr Pat Frankish, Peter Saunders from NAPAC, Paul Williams from Cruse Bereavement Care and Dr Lizzie Ward.

Introduction

The fact that we are all living longer should be something to celebrate. Life expectancy in 1900 was 47 for men and 50 for women and has increased in the intervening century to 78 for men and 82 for women.

It sounds like good news for us all. However, it does mean that the UK, like most highly developed countries, now has a disproportionate number of pensioners. The British Geriatric Society says that in ten years' time, the number of older people will be greater than the number of under-fives, all over the world. By 2033, almost a quarter of the British population is predicted to be over 65, and 5 per cent will be over 85. This means that more and more of us will be responsible for someone who is very elderly and possibly very frail. The NHS already spends 43 per cent of its budget on older people, and more than half of the country's 6 million carers look after an elderly relative.

The question of just *who* will care for all these very old people, and *how* they are best cared for, has still to be addressed. In some cultures, there is said to be no question. Family is family, and the idea of 'abandoning' a loved one in an old people's home is seen as scandalous. It is rather like Victorian Britain where a maiden aunt always seemed to be available to earn her keep by caring for the old, the sick, or children. I once met an elderly lady who had been adopted, as a small child, specifically to act as a companion to her adoptive parents in their old age! So-called 'family' care too often devolves onto women, and women in Britain in the twenty-first century have other responsibilities – careers, mortgages to pay, children and grandchildren to consider. That is not to denigrate male carers – Carers UK says that almost half (42 per cent) of Britain's carers are men.

Living in a three-generation household is not always either practical or desirable. Who cares for Gran or Granddad if you are out at work all day? Is a household of rowdy teenagers really the best place for someone old and sick?

Caring for an elderly parent – or relative or friend – can never be easy. It's hard to see someone you love and care about become older, frailer, less capable and more confused than the person you once knew. And what if your best efforts aren't enough? If the person you're looking after becomes unsettled or unhappy, verbally abusive and angry, blaming you for any difficulties, and refuses to cooperate with family carers or medical and social work professionals? Someone who won't accept help when it's offered, or who insists that you do all the caring, can wreck family relationships and ruin carers' lives.

Some parents become more difficult with age, but there's also the question of the parent who has always been difficult, or where relationships have always been strained. Difficult people don't become easier with age. It's immensely stressful to be responsible for someone who is not only old and frail but also stubborn and cantankerous, who refuses to have 'strangers' in the house, who cancels appointments made by desperate families and insists they can manage alone when this clearly isn't the case.

Here's Rose's story:

> We live in London and my parents live on the Yorkshire coast. We tried to raise the subject of a move as they got older but they refused to consider the idea. We also suggested some home improvements like a downstairs bathroom and a new central heating boiler but they said they didn't want the disruption, even though we were happy to pay.
>
> Their house is damp, poorly insulated, expensive to heat and on a steep hill. It was all right while Dad was still driving but his driving is becoming more and more erratic.
>
> They always insist they are all right but it became clear that they aren't keeping themselves or the house properly clean. They keep ignoring sell-by dates on food and I was convinced they would die of food poisoning. They aren't actually ill, just not quite coping any longer.
>
> Even a neighbour says she is worried about them. We can't keep driving 250 miles to sort them out. I'm an only child so there is no one to help out. Eventually I contacted the local Social Services who were very nice, but Mum was furious and refused to let them in!

If you're nodding in recognition at the problems Rose and her family faced, then this is the book for you. But rest assured. There *is* help out there for older people in today's Britain, even though it might sometimes be difficult to find out about it or access the help you and your relative need.

1

What the problems might be

As you and your parents grow older, your relationship changes in all sorts of subtle ways. Once you relied on them – for help, advice, the occasional loan when money was tight, perhaps babysitting duties when your children were small. Slowly but surely, this changes until you realize that now *you* are responsible for *their* welfare. Sometimes this happens slowly, almost imperceptibly. Sometimes it's sudden, as it was for Veronica.

> I drove down to see my mum and dad in the West Country for a week-end, as I'd often done before. I went in the kitchen door, which was always left unlocked, and said, 'Hi, anyone home?' There was no reply and when I went into the living room there they were, sitting one on either side of the fireplace, fast asleep – at two o'clock in the afternoon! In the old days, they would have heard me driving up and Mum would have had the kettle on before I'd got out of my car. I watched them for a few moments and thought, heavens, these are *old people* now. It was a real shock. Of course, they woke up straight away and were terribly apologetic for dropping off. It didn't matter at all – but that was when I realized that things had changed, and would go on changing.

Lincolnshire-based consultant clinical psychologist Dr Pat Frankish says that everyone, as they move into another stage of life, has to accept a shift in identity, and that this is not always easy.

> The parent who has always been independent and may have helped out their adult child lots of times, finds the shift to being dependent almost intolerable. They can react with irritation and negative behaviour towards their offspring, who they see as having the sort of life *they* used to have.
>
> The adult child in this situation can react with patience and understanding, which may be thrown back at them, or with irritation themselves, leading to a breakdown in the relationship. It falls to the adult child to be tactful and facilitate the illusion of

independence as long as possible. The see-saw swinging the other way, towards the parent being the dependant, takes time to adjust to, but if it is accepted, there is room for a healthy and happy relationship until the parent dies.

The fear of death and dying raises its head and needs to be faced. The time commitment, and the sudden calls to the hospital or the parental home, increase. It is part of the life cycle. Generally speaking, if you have had a good parent/child relationship before the onset of old age, it will continue. If you haven't, it is not going to develop in the position of the caregiver needing care.

Dr Frankish makes a very good point. Any difficulties you have as your parents become older and more dependent have to be seen in the context of the existing relationship you have with them. If it has always been harmonious, there may be less friction between you – although you have to bear in mind that you are still their child and it's just as hard for them to accept the changing circumstances as it is for you!

If your relationship has always been problematic, it's unlikely to get any easier as your parents become more and more dependent. You have a whole lifetime's worth of history, including rows and misunderstandings, or if you're very unlucky, emotional, physical or sexual abuse behind you – what then?

You want to help. You feel you *should* help. They are your parents, after all. (And much the same applies if you are caring for another relative or close friend.) We have all read the harrowing newspaper stories of elderly recluses, found in their homes weeks or even months after their deaths, and wondered, however fleetingly, how their families or 'the authorities' could let it happen. Some people, though, are very hard to help. Here's Anne's experience.

> I tried to get Auntie Lily to plan for a crisis, just in case one came, but she always used to say, 'Let's think about that when it happens.' When she was diagnosed with dementia it was too late, though she then agreed to do anything I wanted. For the previous year, she had said that she didn't need carers, not even once a week to check on her, didn't need a cleaner, certainly wasn't going to arrange power of attorney so that I could take care of her finances for her, didn't want to see the doctor, and was rude to the community psychiatric nurse who used to pop in to check she was all right. She was, in short, bloody difficult.

What might the problems be?

Distance This can be a major issue when you are responsible for older relatives. The days when families grew up, married and grew old in the same geographical area are long gone. Communication may be better than it once was, with fast transport, the Internet, 24/7 telephone connections and Skype, but if your elderly mum has a fall and you live 200 or 2,000 miles away, what can you do? This can cause problems between siblings too, with the members of the family who are near at hand being forced to shoulder most of the burden.

Accommodation The house you grew up in, where your parents may have lived happily for 50 years, may not be in the least suitable for them as they get older. Most family houses aren't. Many older properties only have an upstairs bathroom, which means it's a struggle for older folk to get to the toilet or to enjoy a bath or shower. Older properties also tend to have bigger gardens, which may have been your parents' pride and joy at one time but just mean too much work as they head into later life.

They may live in a country area with no local shop and poor public transport. Being dependent on a car is all very well for fit folk in their fifties and sixties, but country-dwellers can be very isolated in extreme old age. How do they get to the doctor, the dentist, the post office, the podiatrist, the bank?

On the other hand, older people living in the city might not have the same friendly contact with a shifting population of neighbours. They – or you – may feel that they are vulnerable to crime and vandalism (though it's worth remembering that old people are actually far *less* likely to be victims of crime than younger folk: crime against the elderly hits the headlines chiefly because it's rare).

Older people are more at risk of poor health if their home is cold and not properly insulated, or if they are dependent on older, less efficient and more expensive heating systems. They may be concerned about high fuel bills and reluctant to turn on the heating when they need it.

Health Not everyone over 80 is physically and/or mentally infirm, but old age does inevitably bring health concerns. Arthritic joints can make walking, getting up from a chair, getting out of bed, getting into the bath or sitting on the toilet a slow, painful business. Some people are prone to falls, which can lead to serious problems in those whose bones are becoming fragile with age. Chest problems – frequent coughs, colds, virus infections or bronchitis – are also common. Some older folk, especially those living alone, lose interest in food and find preparing meals too much trouble. A healthy, balanced diet and an appropriate exercise regime are just as important for pensioners as they are for younger people, but how many of them really do eat well and get out and about?

Neither can the side effects of common medications be ignored. Many older people have to take drugs to control their angina, asthma, high blood pressure or some other condition. Side effects can include things like stomach upsets, drowsiness, cough or headache. There is also, of course, the possibility that your relative will be diagnosed with a serious illness such as Parkinson's disease, dementia or some form of cancer, all more common in this age group.

Life changes   Few people look forward to getting old – even though it can have its compensations. Retirement offers lots of opportunities to take things easy and to spend time doing what you have always wanted to do, whether that's playing golf all day or visiting the Galapagos Islands. However, it is also an enormous life change. Not everyone reacts well to the idea of no longer being a productive member of society, perhaps feeling 'thrown on the scrap heap' or undervalued. This can lead to depression and may require a lot of psychological adjustment.

Relationships between older couples change too. In 2009, 13,700 couples aged over 60 were granted divorces, and this is the only age group where divorce rates are rising. Perhaps spending 24 hours of the day together when a husband and wife are more used to doing their own thing leads to a strain on a tired marriage. But the risk is there, and again it requires a lot of adjustment. We will look at the issues raised by later-life marriage and stepfamilies in Chapter 9.

Bereavement – the possibility of losing not only one's life partner but also one's oldest and dearest friends – is another by-product of ageing, and can be hard to come to terms with.

Personality clashes   Your relationship with Mum or Dad may always have been a problematic one, and now that you are all older it hasn't got any easier. You may have grown up feeling that you were the least favoured child and been given the impression that you were always a disappointment to one or both of your parents. Perhaps they wanted a boy, or someone to take over the family business, or someone to fulfil all their ambitions at second-hand. What they got was you – an individual who somehow didn't come up to scratch. That's a hard burden to bear.

If you're already being made to feel inadequate and guilty, you can feel worse when your parent, or parents, become older and frailer and hint that what they really want is for you to move back in with them, or for them to move in with you. This can be a particular issue for single middle-aged women but one that can arise for people with families too – as Aileen found out.

> Mum was a real tyrant. If she had moved in with my husband and me he would have left home. She didn't like men much and she disliked him especially, for no apparent reason. She was always having a go and needling him about how much better my sister's husband had done, how much bigger their house was, how much better behaved their children were than ours. The only saving grace was that my sister and I get on very well and I knew that Mum was exactly the same in their house!

We will be looking at ways of dealing with some of these situations in later chapters. However, here are ten 'rules' you should always keep in mind.

1 Your parents have rights – but so do you, and so do the rest of your family. Don't be a martyr.
2 You can't do everything for them, and you shouldn't try. You can only do your best.
3 When it comes to getting help for them, try advising, mentioning, but don't take over.
4 Be tactful and don't patronize them.
5 Retain your sense of humour.
6 Always involve them in any decisions you make about their welfare.
7 Treat them with respect, even when you feel exasperated.
8 Don't impose your standards on them. As long as they are warm and comfortable it doesn't matter if their home doesn't have every mod con.

9   Some people respond better to suggestions from a contemporary (an old friend?) or an authority figure (the doctor?) than they do from their own family.
10 Remember, you will be old yourself one day. How would *you* like to be treated?

Planning ahead

As with any relationship, open and honest communication can be tremendously helpful. One of the things that older people dislike most – and we'll be exploring this in the next chapter – is the feeling that *they are no longer in control of their lives*. If you, and they, make some plans in advance, or at least talk about them, they will feel that they have made their own decisions about their care, and that can only be a good thing.

Of course, you need to be tactful when bringing up the subject. You might, for example, offer to mow the lawn when you're visiting them and say, afterwards, something like, 'Phew! I'm worn out, Dad! How on earth do you manage to keep the garden looking so good?' That gives your father a chance to say that he is, in fact, finding it much harder work than he once did, and you might then suggest he gets someone in to help with the tougher jobs.

A stay in hospital, or even perhaps a doctor's appointment, could be a blessing in disguise. The hospital has a duty to arrange for care in patients' homes after they come out, and a 'care package' could include aids such as grab rails or a commode. Remember that some older people are much more receptive to helpful suggestions from an authority figure like the doctor, as Philip's mother was.

> She had very bad arthritis in her knees and although she lived in a ground-floor flat and I was on hand to help, she was walking less and less. Even getting to the bathroom was a struggle and she had a few accidents. I kept telling her that she should do as much walking as she could, even around the flat, or she would lose the use of her legs altogether, but she wouldn't listen. Then she developed a chest infection, and while she was in hospital she was treated by a very nice young doctor. He said exactly the same thing to her about walking and she fluttered her eyelashes at him and said, 'Yes, doctor!' I had to bite my tongue . . . but his advice did the trick!

Any life changes coming up can be presented in a positive light, too. Instead of suggesting that your parents can no longer cope with the house they're living in, it could help to point out the advantages of moving to a smaller and more manageable property. They could, for instance:

- be nearer to you and the rest of the family;
- be nearer to friends, shops, the doctor and other facilities;
- be much less dependent on the car;
- free up some of their capital to spend on something they would enjoy.

There are huge advantages to thinking ahead, both for you and for your parents. If you wait for a crisis, such as a sudden breakdown in their health, decisions may have to be made quickly and fewer options may be available. Depending on where you live and what sort of accommodation is needed, there may be waiting lists for sheltered housing or places in the most attractive and convenient care homes. These are all options that can – indeed should – be considered well before they are needed, so that the right choices can be made and your parents feel that they are still in control, as Patricia's parents do.

My brothers and I were surprised when Mum and Dad told us they had decided to move from their village house into the nearest town two miles away, where there was a very nice block of sheltered flats. They were around 80 but in very good health, Dad was still driving and they both rode into town on their bikes to do the shopping!

They said they had been discussing the issue with their friends, most of whom were around the same age, and had decided that this was the best choice for them. My brothers and I all live more than 100 miles away, so 'popping in' to keep an eye on them wasn't an option. They had lived in their house for 20 years, so it was quite an upheaval but we all helped and they never looked back. The new flat was much smaller, but all on one level, with a lift and nice communal gardens they could enjoy. They were just behind the High Street so shopping was easy, and there was a good social life in the flats so they made a lot of new friends.

We were pleased they'd decided to move although there had been absolutely no pressure from us.

2

Coping with feelings about changes in later life

On the whole, care homes for old and frail people or those suffering from dementia do not get a good press. The image of an 'old people's home' is too often of elderly residents slumped in chairs around an unwatched TV screen. As is often the case in the media, it's the scandals and examples of dreadful mistreatment that hit the headlines, not the well-run homes where residents are cared for and encouraged to enjoy outings, social events, art classes and visits from friends and family.

In the world of professional care, the current buzzwords are 'person-centred care', and the best care homes are run on this principle, which was pioneered by Professor Tom Kitwood in the 1990s. He was looking at dementia care in particular, but the principles involved are the same and are true even for people who are cared for at home or by friends and family.

Person-centred care means treating the person as you would want to be treated yourself, and focusing on them as an individual rather than just a 'case'. A recent report by the NHS and the Age UK charity, 'Dignity in Care', made common-sense recommendations about the way older patients are treated in hospital and care homes. The report complains about the way very old people are often seen – as a burden on the NHS and families, as incapable and dependent. Sometimes they are referred to, insultingly, as 'bed-blockers' simply because the right out-of-hospital care is not always provided for them.

One care group ran a special training programme for their staff to give them some insight into how it feels to be old, frail and cared for. They weren't called by their own names, they were left alone for long periods with nothing to do, they were brought cups of sweet tea when they had asked for unsweetened coffee, and generally treated as if they didn't matter. The programme was an eye-opener for those staff members, and offers lessons for anyone who is caring for an old and sometimes difficult parent.

Try and put yourself in your relative's place. *How do you think they feel?*

Fortunately, some research has been done into just how older people *do* feel about the care they are offered, and why it might be refused. Your parents may not just be being 'difficult'. They might have genuine reservations. A project at the Department of Sociological Studies, University of Sheffield, found that older people need to see themselves, and to be seen, not as dependent service users but as whole persons, with lives of value and achievement.

Older people may refuse help for various reasons:

- They don't want to admit that they can no longer cope alone and want to stay independent, however unrealistic this might be.
- They are afraid of losing the abilities that they still have.
- To some extent they too share the negative attitudes to old age that are all too common in society.

They might express opinions such as:

- old people's homes are for people who are confused, or for those whose families don't care about them;
- day centres aren't for people like us;
- home care is for lazy people;
- I/we don't want to live with a lot of old people.

Could this be true of your mum and dad? Interestingly, this research also suggested that 'care providers' – which could mean you – should *expect* some resistance from the old people. Consultant clinical psychologist Dr Pat Frankish says:

Some older people who are hard to help would have been hard to help before they became old. People who are fiercely independent have a fear of being controlled by others. This will usually stem from experiences in childhood when they have had things taken away, or had things done that they didn't like. Deciding that you don't need anyone else is a defence and works reasonably well until infirmity sets in. At that point, their whole identity as an independent person is threatened, and this leads to anger and frustration. It is not possible to feel grateful to someone for helping you if your core feeling is resentment of the fact that help is necessary. If possible, we need to find ways to help without it showing, and certainly without expecting thanks or gratitude.

A more recent study of well-being in older people was carried out at the University of Brighton in conjunction with Age UK and the results were published in April 2012. The researchers, Professor Marian Barnes and Dr Lizzie Ward, found that isolation and loneliness were major issues for the very old, because of loss of mobility, confidence and bereavement, as you would expect.

They also found that older people often found it hard to acknowledge that they needed support, and were sometimes reluctant to ask for help because of a mixture of pride and embarrassment. They felt that carers – whether family or professionals – could help by:

- listening carefully to what the old person was saying and responding appropriately;
- allowing them to make their own decisions about the services they accepted;
- giving them time, acknowledging their feelings, building up trust, and being consistent and reliable.

The researchers said that families are important to older people, but that 'not wanting to be a burden' was a common theme. Families, they said, 'could involve difficult and painful relationships, distance and estrangement'. The loss of long-term friends was very strongly felt and everyday interactions with good neighbours and even 'familiar strangers' in local shops were important to older people's well-being.

Old people in other similar surveys spoke about the importance of 'not giving up', 'not letting yourself go', and enjoying being able to give, as well as get, support from their families. Brian, whose elderly parents live nearby, says that he has noticed this.

Mum and Dad are in their eighties and frail, though they manage quite well. My wife and I have noticed how much brighter they seem when they have something they can do for us. For example, if we go away for a weekend or a holiday, they are keen for us to have a meal, or coffee and sandwiches, with them when we get back, to save us the trouble of cooking. They like to come in and feed the cats for us, too.

There seems to be some stigma involved in asking for help from the Social Services and an assumption that such help is only available for the very poor. Many people simply have no idea about the amount of help, both practical and financial, that is available and don't know where or how to access it. Some are put off by the bureaucracy of 'having to fill in a lot of forms' and the perceived indignity of 'strangers poking their noses into my business'.

What can family carers learn from all this? Caring for anyone, however difficult they might be, is made a lot easier if you make a genuine effort to put yourself in their place. Imagine how it might be to be very old, unable to do a lot of the things that once made up your life, and perhaps being the sole survivor of a long and happy marriage, or a crowd of friends. Here's Jim's story.

> I'm 93 now and my wife Marjorie is 92. We live in a sheltered flat about a mile from our son and daughter-in-law. For our age, we don't think we do badly. I'm becoming very deaf and although I have a hearing aid and have been backwards and forwards to audiologists it doesn't seem to help much. I'm all right talking on a one-to-one basis but in a crowd it's hopeless and I do feel rather cut off.
>
> I used to be a sportsman in my younger days, at school and in the Army, and played badminton and learned judo after that. Now I have a bad back and it's as much as I can do to get out of bed in the morning. I get tired, too, and like a nap after lunch. Until recently Marje and I went for a walk to the local park every day, but her knees are bad now so we have been confined to the flat and grounds.
>
> I can see Marje getting more and more frail and forgetful. Our GP referred her to a memory clinic and she has been prescribed tablets but I'm not sure what they are. Our children are very good, and our grandchildren and great-grandchildren come to visit, but we miss our old friends. I had three schoolfriends I used to go for pub lunches with but they've all died off and I'm the last one left.
>
> Marje and I both sometimes say that we have lived too long.

Thinking of your parent as an individual, and imagining how they might feel, can really help you to understand that when they seem to be being awkward and uncooperative, they may actually be feeling . . . what? Frightened of what the future holds for them, when the opportunities it presents seem more and more limited? Humiliated, because dads who used to be breadwinners and took the responsibility for their families have to get used to the idea of themselves as helpless old men, and mums who used to be the family carers are now the cared for? Frustrated, because easy jobs they once took for granted, from getting up and dressed in the morning to walking to the paper shop or the supermarket, are now beyond their reach? Lonely and unhappy, because every telephone call or piece of news from friends and contemporaries seems to feature illness, disability and death?

The chances are that they don't mean to take these feelings of misery and frustration out on you. It's just that you're nearest! You may sometimes be able to deflect their frustrations, however.

Suggest practical solutions. For example, an enormous amount of equipment is available that is designed to make life easier for older and disabled people, from wheelchairs and electric buggies to gadgets to help them pull socks or stockings on. We look at some of these in detail in Chapter 8. Even frail oldies don't need to be housebound.

Talk to them about friends they have lost. 'Reminiscence therapy' is often used by old-age psychologists and care workers to act as a kind of 'keep fit' for the mind. Old photos, movies, CDs of popular songs or magazines picked up for pence at a car boot sale can inspire even older people with short-term memory problems. If you, and their other relatives like grandchildren, take a genuine interest in their lives and memories, it can help to make them feel valued. Ask them how they met their oldest friend or their spouse. Grandchildren could ask them what teenage life, fashion, music was like when they were young. Today's teens, glued to their mobile phones 24/7, can be fascinated to realize that a couple of generations ago many households didn't even have landlines!

Encourage them in their hobbies and interests – either the ones they have always had, or new ones, sometimes even surprising ones! An old lady I once knew said the highlight of her week was going swimming with her nine-year-old granddaughter and her friends. My Great-Aunt Annie adored visiting the local primary school to talk to the children about playground games before the last war.

Once they have got over their initial resistance, the world of the Internet can open up new horizons for them, as well as saving them time and effort spent on things like shopping. Age UK has a Digital Inclusion Network scheme to introduce older people to computer use with jargon-free courses. You can find out more about this from the

Age UK helpline or website (see Useful addresses). Or perhaps they would like to make a 'memory book' – a scrapbook full of old photos and notes – as a family heirloom to be passed on to the grandchildren or great-grandchildren?

3

Mental distress in later life

Caring for older people can be made easier if you are able to put yourself in their position, and realize that, far from trying to be awkward, they are actually suffering from genuine distress. Knowing this doesn't mean that you will never find their behaviour and reactions exasperating, but it does help you to stand back, take a deep breath and work out what the problem really is.

In the previous chapter we looked at feelings, and some of the most obvious reasons why old people might feel depressed, from social factors such as bereavement, isolation and boredom, to illness and painful chronic conditions like arthritis for which no real cure is currently available. Mental distress – and specifically its most common forms, depression and anxiety – is very widespread in later life.

Depression

It is said that depression is the most common mental health problem in older people and is the underlying reason why many over-seventies visit their GP. Sometimes it can be hard for older folk, who are less used than younger generations to openness about their feelings, to admit that they're feeling depressed. This is a generation that prided itself on being strong and stoical and 'just getting on with things'. Small wonder that it's hard for them to let down their guard and admit that they are feeling down.

It isn't surprising that older people may feel depressed. Their reasons for developing the condition may be social or they may be physical. They may be depressed because they are ill or in pain, increasingly disabled and feeling 'cut off' or marginalized from society. They may be lonely and isolated with little contact with others. They may be suffering from the side effects of prescription drugs. Beta-blockers, for example, prescribed to treat angina and other heart disorders, blood pressure drugs, steroids used to control inflammation, and sedatives, can all cause depression in some users. If this turns out to be the case, alternative treatments are often available.

The life changes we discussed in previous chapters, such as retirement or bereavement, can also be factors in the development of depression. Just feeling that the best years of your life are far behind you and that there's little to look forward to can trigger depression in some susceptible people.

Symptoms

The symptoms of depression in older people may not differ very much from those in younger folk. Apart from the obvious – a general feeling of misery – they can include:

- loss of interest and pleasure in life, even in things they previously enjoyed;
- feelings of uselessness and guilt, especially if they are being cared for – all the reports on depression in older people mention 'not wanting to be a burden' on family and friends as a big worry for those who are old and frail;
- poor concentration and lack of energy;
- reduced appetite and weight loss;
- sleep problems.

You can see that sometimes all these symptoms *could* be seen as just the result of getting older, but that's not always the case. If you notice your elderly parents complaining of any of the above symptoms, you could suggest, gently, that a visit to the GP could be in order. Just as old people don't have to be housebound because they're physically frail, they don't *have* to be unhappy and depressed either. Help is available and depression can be treated.

Other causes of depression

Why some people – old or young – get depression and others don't is not known. Researchers have not yet found a gene that could 'cause' depression, but it's believed that there is a genetic element involved in the condition. It also appears that depression could be the result of an imbalance of the chemicals in the brain. Antidepressant drugs work by correcting some of these imbalances. However, that doesn't explain *why* some people get depressed. As well as problems in the present, such as bereavement or illness, unhappy experiences from a person's past, even going back to childhood, can make a person more likely to experience depression. Older people who are ill, who have lost interest in preparing and eating meals and are therefore missing out on vital nutrients, are also at greater risk of becoming depressed. Vitamin B12 and folic acid deficiency are both linked to depressive illness, so it is especially important that elderly people continue to eat a healthy, balanced diet with plenty of fruit and vegetables.

Getting a diagnosis

It's very important that depression in older people is correctly diagnosed, because it can be confused with other conditions, such as dementia. The relationship between the two conditions is complicated because people who actually have dementia may be depressed as well! However, while dementia is a progressive condition (see Chapter 5) for which no cure is currently available, older people can be successfully treated for depression.

Dementia is a brain disorder. Depression is a mood disorder. Forgetfulness, an inability to concentrate, apathy, lack of interest in normal activities and sadness can be symptoms of either dementia or depression. However, a person with depression:

- will know the time, the date, and where he or she is – someone with dementia may not;
- will be able to speak, write and get around normally, even if he is slow and not very interested in doing so – dementia may affect all these skills;
- will be aware of becoming forgetful and will be worried about it – someone with dementia may not notice any short-term memory problems, but if she does, she will not be particularly concerned.

Treatment for depression

It's in the nature of the illness to believe that nothing can be done that will make you feel better! Somehow, if your elderly mum or dad is depressed, you have to persuade them that they can be helped. You can't roll back the years for them, or bring back friends and loved ones they have lost, but you *can* make sure that everything possible is being done to enable them to make the most of the life they have.

Some of the ways in which this can be done are actually quite simple – and useful for the sort of person who 'doesn't want to bother the doctor' or 'doesn't want to take a lot of tablets'. Mild depression can often be helped by keeping occupied. Hobbies, interests and visits from family and friends can help here. Exercise and keeping fit are known to help lift the spirits, and you don't have to be a marathon runner – a walk in the fresh air can release 'feel-good' hormones in the brain and improve a person's mood. Many local authorities and gyms offer exercise and dance classes especially for older people which your parent might enjoy.

Remember the importance of a healthy diet too. Even older people with small appetites can benefit from fresh, tasty, well-prepared food. Grilled meat or fish with vegetables or a baked potato with a cheese or tuna-and-sweetcorn filling, accompanied by a salad, are all nutritious and easy to prepare. Folate, found in green vegetables, beetroot, black-eye beans and peanuts, and its synthetic form, folic acid, found in fortified breakfast cereals, is also said to boost low mood.

MIND, the mental health charity (see Useful addresses), says that the relationship between diet and mental and emotional health is a complicated one. Caffeine, for instance, which is found in tea and chocolate drinks as well as coffee, can give a quick energy boost, but too much can make some people feel nervous and jumpy. For optimum mental health, a 'feel-good' diet should include:

- six to eight glasses of water a day;
- five or more portions of fruit and vegetables every day;
- a healthy breakfast to start the day;
- regular mealtimes so that blood sugar levels don't vary wildly – this can help to avoid mood swings;
- food that releases energy slowly, such as oats and wholegrains, rather than sweets, cakes and biscuits;
- essential fatty acids, especially Omega-3, the kind found in oily fish, which are good for the brain;
- nuts and seeds, which contain a lot of useful nutrients.

It can be hard to persuade stubborn older people to change their diets. Introducing changes slowly is the most tactful way to do it. On the other hand, your parents probably come from a generation that prided itself on 'proper' home-cooked meat-and-two-veg dinners rather than today's tins, packets and takeaways; traditional meals can be made healthier by substituting semi-skimmed for full-cream milk, using low-fat dairy products, grilling rather than frying, and replacing stodgy puddings with fresh fruit.

Antidepressant drugs may be prescribed to help lift depression in older people, just as they are for younger folk. They may have side effects, or interact with other medication that your parent may be taking, and all this should be discussed with the doctor before a drug is prescribed. They work by raising the levels of neurotransmitters in the brain, and it will take about two weeks before improvements are noticed. The prescribing GP will tell you how long they need to be taken for. As with all medication, it's important for your parent to complete the course and not stop taking them when he or she begins to feel better, in case the symptoms return.

Antidepressant drugs commonly prescribed include:

- SSRIs (selective serotonin reuptake inhibitors), such as Prozac or Seroxat
- TCAs (tricyclic antidepressants), such as Anafranil or Tofranil
- MAOIs (monoamine oxydase inhibitors), prescribed for those who are anxious as well as depressed and who suffer from phobias. They are less commonly used today because they interact with many foods, such as cheese, yeast extract, or red wine.

People suffering from depression may also be helped by what are known as 'talking therapies', such as CBT (cognitive behavioural therapy), instead of, or in addition to, antidepressant medication. Psychotherapy or counselling may benefit some people – if you can persuade your parent that talking over their feelings with a stranger would benefit them! You can find out more from the GP. There are also self-help groups, both 'real-life' and on the Internet, such as Depression UK (see Useful addresses). Sharing worries anonymously with other people who have been through, or are going through, the same thing can be therapeutic.

There are many complementary therapies that are said to help with depression. Among the herbal remedies sometimes used in this way is St John's wort. If you and your parent are interested in exploring these alternatives, make sure you consult a reputable practitioner who is a member of the National Institute of Medical Herbalists (see Useful addresses). St John's wort may interact with conventional antidepressant medication, so it's important that the GP knows your parent is considering taking it. Other complementary treatments that may prove useful include aromatherapy, in which the therapist chooses specially selected essential oils to be used in a massage, in the bath, or in a burner to improve mood and give a heightened sense of well-being.

'Pet therapy' is also recommended for lifting mood. If your parent is fond of animals, contact with a dog or cat can be both soothing and uplifting. Many animal charities organize pet therapy visits to old people in care and nursing homes.

Anxiety

Like depression, anxiety is common in older people, but that doesn't mean that it's an inevitable part of getting older, or that it can't be successfully treated. As people become more frail they face physical challenges and it becomes harder and harder to do simple things they once took for granted, like climbing stairs or getting into or out of the bath. It takes only a minor slip or fall to worry them, making them concerned and anxious about the same thing happening again – or something worse. That's often where anxiety begins. Older people can become worried about going outside their 'comfort zone'. Inevitably, if they feel this way, their lives become more and more restricted and this in itself can increase their anxiety.

Everyone gets anxious from time to time. You don't have to be a frail old person to feel nervous about, for instance, a long flight to an unfamiliar country, or a medical procedure. A little nervous anticipation is normal and natural and doesn't have to be a problem. It's only when anxiety seems to take over someone's life that help might be needed to deal with it. There are several different forms of anxiety, including the following types.

- **Generalized anxiety disorder**, where the symptoms of anxiety (see below) are experienced in a general way and for no apparent reason. People with GAD find they feel tense, restless or worried most of the time, and afraid of things that *might* happen, without being able to explain exactly what they are worried about. Some older people feel self-conscious when they first begin to use a walking aid – perhaps a stick, or a frame – or if they need to use a wheelchair. Outings can be a source of anxiety for an older person if she is not sure where the toilets are, or whether she will be able to get there in time when she needs to go. Tactful questioning can provide reassurance about that.

- **Phobias**. A phobia is an intense, disproportionate fear of a particular object or situation, which is so severe that it affects everyday life. Common phobias include claustrophobia (fear of confined spaces), agoraphobia (fear of leaving the safety of home) and social phobias, where you fear being around other people because of worries about what they think of you. There are also single-issue phobias, such as being afraid of flying, or of spiders, or of hospitals.
- **Panic attacks**. These are sudden, extremely intense attacks of anxiety, often coming on 'out of the blue'. The anxiety experienced is so severe that the person may be convinced he is going to faint, collapse, or even have a heart attack and die.
- **OCD** (obsessive–compulsive disorder), which is when someone becomes obsessed with her own, often frightening, thoughts, and devises rituals (like repeated hand-washing or going back time after time to check she has switched the lights off) in order to be able to cope.
- **PTSD** (post-traumatic stress disorder), which affects people who have been through a difficult or traumatic experience, and relive what happened in their minds over and over again, finding it impossible to 'move on'.

Causes of anxiety

The causes of anxiety can be similar to the causes of depression. An upsetting or traumatic experience may make one person feel depressed and another anxious, depending on their personality and also their past experiences. Some people are just natural worriers, or may have learned to react anxiously over the years. Anxiety can be a vicious circle, as it has so many physical symptoms (see below). Your parent may be so worried about heart palpitations that he or she becomes even more anxious, which causes more severe heart palpitations – and so on. Being lonely, bored, isolated or bereaved can also trigger anxiety in susceptible people.

Symptoms of anxiety

Anxiety is the body's way of responding to a situation that seems frightening or threatening. It is sometimes known as the 'fight or flight' response because the body prepares itself to either fight the threat, or run away from it. Muscles tense up ready for action. Stress hormones like adrenaline and cortisol pour into the bloodstream. The heart beats faster and the breathing rate increases. Animals depend on this response for their survival in the wild and human reactions are just the same, even though in reality there may be nothing to be afraid of. Anxious people will feel a mixture of physical and psychological symptoms, for example:

- heart palpitations, shortness of breath, sweating, dry mouth, butterflies in the stomach, dizziness, shaking, aches and pains, nausea, diarrhoea, sleeping problems;
- worry, restlessness, irritability, an edgy feeling, poor sleep, sometimes confusion and difficulty in concentrating.

Treatments for anxiety

Some of the drugs and therapies used to treat depression are also used to relieve anxiety. Self-help techniques can also be useful. Even something as simple as a brisk walk, a favourite meal, or a chat with a sympathetic friend or family member can help. Controlled, regular breathing, rather than hyperventilating and taking in great gulps of air, can be a useful skill to learn. So is distraction – soothing the panicky feelings by concentrating on something else, like counting the number of red cars that pass in the street, or singing a favourite song under your breath. If they are allowed to, the panicky feelings do die away.

Support groups for sufferers from anxiety and phobias include Anxiety Care UK and No Panic (see Useful addresses). Knowing that other people have learned to manage their anxious feelings can be very reassuring.

Relaxation techniques, such as meditation, yoga, t'ai chi (known as 'meditation in motion') and autogenic training, can relieve anxiety and are suitable for all age groups. CDs and DVDs of soothing music and guided relaxation are widely available. Different types of meditation can help people to achieve a state of deep and complete relaxation, which benefits both an anxious mind and a tense body. Yoga – the name is derived from a Sanskrit word meaning 'union' – has been practised for thousands of years. A combination of controlled breathing and physical movement promotes union between mind and body. T'ai chi is a Chinese therapy, especially popular among older Chinese people, which combines gentle exercise with meditation and is useful for reducing anxiety. Autogenic training, devised by a German doctor in the 1920s and introduced into Britain in the 1970s, involves learning a set of very simple, repetitive instructions; when practised regularly, these calm both mind and body, promote total relaxation, and improve sleep. (See Useful addresses for contact details to obtain more information on these therapies.)

Drugs, including some of the antidepressants mentioned in the previous section, can be helpful in reducing anxiety. Other anti-anxiety drugs that may be prescribed include benzodiazepines (Valium), which are very effective in treating anxiety but should be used for no more than two weeks as they can be addictive; and anxiolytics (buspirone), which work in a similar way to Valium but are not addictive. These can take up to two weeks to start working, so it's important to take the tablets according to the doctor's instructions. Alcohol and grapefruit juice can react with this drug, so they should be avoided.

Talking therapies like counselling, psychotherapy or cognitive behavioural therapy can be useful in treating anxiety. Phobias, for instance, are often tackled with a mixture of relaxation techniques and de-sensitization. People afraid of spiders may be taught to relax, and then shown a photo of a spider, gradually learning that if they remain relaxed they can look at, and eventually even touch, a spider without panicking.

4

Other mental health problems

Like everyone else, older people can sometimes be mentally ill. If you are trying to care for a parent who, earlier in their life, was diagnosed with a serious mental illness such as schizophrenia or bipolar disorder (once better known as manic depression) you could find yourself facing particular challenges. These conditions are much rarer than anxiety, depression or dementia (we will be looking at dementia in Chapter 5) and are outside the scope of this book, as they are most commonly diagnosed in people in their twenties and thirties.

Mental illnesses

Schizophrenia is the most common serious mental illness, affecting about 1 in every 100 people in Britain. People with schizophrenia do not have a 'split personality', nor are they necessarily dangerous or aggressive. In fact they are more likely to be the victims of crime than the perpetrators, and they are far more likely to harm themselves than hurt other people.

Symptoms of schizophrenia include hallucinations, false beliefs, agitation and strange behaviour, and additionally low mood, lack of motivation, withdrawal from social activity and relationships. Treatment is with a mixture of psychiatric care, including in-patient hospital treatment on occasions, social rehabilitation and anti-psychotic drugs. These drugs are divided into 'typicals', an older type of drug, such as haloperidol, which can be effective but can also cause troublesome side effects, and 'atypicals', such as risperidone and olanzapine, which are generally preferred by patients because they cause fewer side effects.

There is a condition known as late onset schizophrenia which affects a very few older people. It seems to be a controversial issue among psychiatrists who don't always agree on what 'late onset' actually means; and sometimes a condition appearing in the over-sixties is referred to as 'very late onset' schizophrenia.

Bipolar disorder is another condition most commonly diagnosed in young people. Symptoms include extreme mood swings, with severe highs and lows and often stable periods in between. People diagnosed as bipolar may also experience delusions and hallucinations. They are usually treated with medication that helps them to manage their symptoms, principally lithium, which needs to be carefully monitored because long-term use can cause kidney or thyroid problems. People with bipolar disorder may also be treated with anti-psychotic drugs.

If your parent has been treated for either of these conditions, the most useful thing you can do is work with them and the mental health team caring for them, which could include their GP, a local community psychiatric nurse and/or a psychiatrist. MIND, the mental health charity, recommends that carers shouldn't try to argue a mentally ill person out of their delusions, nor pretend to share them. Instead, try to empathize with the way they are feeling.

If you don't feel the person you're caring for is getting a fair deal, you might think of contacting a local advocacy service. Independent advocates work on behalf of vulnerable people – who may be old, have mental health issues, or both – to ensure that they are enabled to speak out, express their views and defend their rights. An advocate will represent their wishes without judging them or putting forward their own opinion.

You can find out about advocacy schemes from Action for Advocacy or the Older People's Advocacy Alliance. More information about mental illness and how the mentally ill can be helped can be obtained from MIND, Re-Think and Bipolar UK (all contact details in Useful addresses).

Personality disorders

Psychiatry is a medical field that is always evolving, and conditions that in the past might have been passed off as 'Uncle Fred's eccentricity' are now being given medical labels, such as 'borderline personality disorder'. What looks to other people like challenging behaviour could be the result of this kind of condition. Personality disorders tend to be under-diagnosed, and mental health charities sometimes say that the label is misunderstood and makes people feel stigmatized.

Most of us find that as we mature we can vary our behaviour and our reactions to others according to our circumstances, and so manage to cope effectively with life. People with personality disorders find this hard. Their range of attitudes and emotions is limited; other people tend to avoid them and they may become quite isolated.

Personality disorders usually become obvious during adolescence or young adulthood. There are several different 'types' and all can, of course, vary in severity. Someone with borderline personality disorder may have mood swings and be very impulsive and prone to self-harming behaviour. Someone diagnosed as obsessive–compulsive may be a controlling type who wants everything to be perfect. Someone with dependent personality disorder may come across as more than normally weak and needy. A person with 'narcissistic' traits can seem exceptionally self-centred.

Those who in the past might have been described as psychopaths are now often diagnosed with anti-social personality disorder. While most people with a personality disorder are neither violent nor a danger to others, 'anti-social' types may become involved in criminal activity or be drawn to overuse of drink or drugs.

Since 2003, according to MIND, there has been a 'Knowledge and Understanding' framework to train mental health professionals to work with those with personality disorders, which are thought to be difficult to treat. Good relationships with trusted health professionals, and group and individual therapies can be helpful. Drugs can be used to treat some of the associated problems like depression. Carers need to realize that those with personality disorders can also be intelligent, creative and likeable, and that the best you can do for them is to make sure that they are getting the help they need from the mental health services.

Autistic spectrum disorders

Like personality disorders, autistic spectrum disorders such as Asperger's syndrome often went unrecognized in the past, so older people might never have received an accurate diagnosis. These disorders affect the way a person relates to, and communicates with, the rest of the world, and once again they can vary in severity. Asperger's syndrome, for example, was only identified 50 years ago. According to the Asperger's Foundation (see Useful addresses), those affected (more commonly men and boys) are often of above average intelligence, honest, reliable and determined. However, they can also seem aloof, uninterested in other people, preferring their own company, and sometimes have unusual mannerisms and obsessive interests – which can often explain Uncle Fred's eccentricities!

(Officially, as of May 2013 the term 'Asperger's syndrome' is being dropped from the revised fifth edition of the Diagnostic and Statistical Manual of Mental Disorders (DSM-5), and being replaced by 'autism spectrum disorder'. This is a controversial decision, and in practice the name Asperger has become so entrenched in popular and psychological culture – even to the abbreviation 'Aspie' – that it's unlikely to disappear.)

Alcohol problems in older people

Schizophrenia, as we have seen, is the most common serious mental illness, affecting about 1 person in 100. According to the Royal College of Physicians, however, as many as *one in six* older men in this country may be drinking enough alcohol to cause harm. The figure for older women is something like 1 in 15.

Drinking alcohol is so firmly established as part of the way we live that it's fantastically difficult to get people to admit that they might have a drink problem. Most of us drink occasionally. Most of us are not harmed by our drinking and there's some evidence that moderate drinking can actually be beneficial. It's important to remember, though, that alcohol is a powerful drug and like all drugs it can be harmful if misused.

For some reason, older people seem especially reluctant to take safe drinking messages on board. In June 2011, the BBC reported on a study by the Royal College of Physicians that suggested that the healthy drinking limits for adults, currently set at 14 units a week for women and 21 for men, should be halved for those over 65. A maximum of 1.5 units a day was suggested.

This provoked a furious response from the 'Saga generation', with complaints about the 'nanny state' and remarks like 'eating, drinking and going to the pub are among the few pleasures remaining to us'. Can drinking too much *really* be such a problem for Britain's pensioners? And could it be affecting someone you care for?

The figures are pretty startling. There has been a 62 per cent increase in the number of hospital admissions for alcohol-related illness in those aged over 65. More people in this age group than 16- to 24-year-olds are admitted to hospital for alcohol-related reasons. When we think of problem drinkers we imagine violent young men brandishing cans of strong lager, or mini-skirted young women staggering home from nightclubs, rather than OAPs.

Here's what Sir Ian Gilmore, Chair of the UK Alcohol Health Alliance, had to say in the summer of 2012:

> Contrary to the public perception that alcohol abuse is more of a problem for young people, the media and political focus on young binge-drinkers has effectively overshadowed the problems for older drinkers – hidden drinkers suffering hidden diseases. Older drinkers suffer from different medical conditions that are not always identified as being due to alcohol – for example cancers, and hypertension. These diseases are strongly linked to alcohol use.

Part of the problem seems to be that older people who may always have enjoyed going to the pub or having wine with their meals simply don't realize that the effects of alcohol become both stronger and longer lasting with age. For example, as we age our bodies tend to lose muscle, gain fat and break down alcohol more slowly. Our reactions become slower and our balance worse. Often, health problems that are thought of as 'just down to old age', such as falls, memory loss, confusion, or shaking limbs, may be signs of a drinking problem. GPs tend not to ask older patients about their drinking, and older drinkers themselves may feel ashamed or embarrassed, or simply be unaware that they can no longer drink the same amount as they could when they were younger.

Drinking too much can affect older people's health in many ways, from the relatively minor, such as headaches and upset stomachs, to the more serious. It can make many later-life health issues worse. It increases the risk of accidents of all kinds, incontinence, coronary heart disease, high blood pressure, strokes, poor sleep, osteoporosis, various kinds of cancer and dementia. It can affect people in ways they might not think of. For example, it can be tempting for older folk to have a tot of rum or brandy to warm themselves up, but alcohol actually speeds up the loss of body heat, so in cold weather or a cold house, in extreme cases, hypothermia could result. Alcohol is a diuretic, so if you drink a lot you need to go to the toilet more often, which could lead to dehydration.

Some people, whether old or young, might argue that it's no one's business but their own how much they drink, but that's never strictly true. It's been estimated that elderly car drivers are three times more likely to be involved in an accident after even a small amount of alcohol than those who don't drink. People who smoke as well as drink are at particular risk – they may drift off to sleep after a few drinks without putting their cigarettes out properly, perhaps causing house fires. Al-Anon, the charity for the friends and families of drinkers, makes the point that each problem drinker affects the lives of five or six other people, including family and carers.

Another very important point is that alcohol can have very different effects when it's combined with prescription drugs. Since about eight out of ten older people take prescribed drugs, according to the Royal College of Physicians, drug interactions can be a big issue. About one-third of the elderly, according to some figures, are on four different types of medication, which makes the risks of combining them with alcohol even higher. Alcohol adds to the effect of sleeping tablets, for instance, but reduces the efficiency of warfarin, the blood-thinning drug prescribed to prevent blood clots. It makes sense when a GP prescribes almost any drug to check whether it's safe to drink alcohol during the course of medication.

Why older people drink

Drinking may just be habit. If your dad's social life has always centred round the local pub, the golf clubhouse or a working men's club, the chances are that drinking has been a part of it. If your parents have always enjoyed a bottle of wine with dinner or a gin and tonic to start the evening, they may very well resist the idea of any change.

Drinking can be a response to stress, just as it can in younger people. All the life changes we discussed in Chapter 2, from retirement to isolation and bereavement, can make people look for solutions. Sometimes, sadly, the solution they choose is alcohol.

How you can help

Awareness is the first step to helping with your parent's drink problem. If you know he or she has always been a drinker and you notice that their health is deteriorating in some of the ways mentioned above – an increase in falls, shakiness, confusion, perhaps incontinence – you should consider alcohol as a possible cause.

It is *never* easy to suggest to anyone that they might be drinking too much, whether that person is a friend of your own age or a much-loved elderly relative. People can be extremely defensive about their drinking. A BBC *Panorama* programme in 2012, fronted by presenter Joan Bakewell, looked at drinking problems in older people. It emerged from interviews that old people particularly dislike being 'told what to do' – and what *not* to do! And a common reaction to health warnings about drinking was, 'Why worry, when you're old already?'

Al-Anon, the charity that supports the families and friends of problem drinkers, underlines the fact that no one can stop another person drinking unless that person wants to stop. Telling Dad or Mum to give up alcohol, especially if the pub, the club or the Bingo represents their main social life, is likely to be counter-productive. Most drinkers, and also those who have decided to give up alcohol, say that lecturing, cajoling, badgering, disapproving or criticizing are a waste of time. Does that mean that there is nothing a relative or carer can do to help?

The charity Drink Aware (see Useful addresses) says that such a delicate conversation should be approached with sensitivity and empathy, and it is best to show concern, not disapproval. Remain as calm as you can, don't be judgemental or sound angry, and use 'I' language rather than 'you' language (which tends to sound accusing). In other words, it's better to say, 'I've noticed you're drinking more these days, what do you think?' or, 'I'm worried because you seem to be having a lot of falls/tummy upsets/blackouts – do you think you could be drinking a bit too much?' rather than, 'You're drinking too much, Dad!'

Be prepared for your parent to be angry, defensive, insulted or to feel upset and humiliated. Don't argue, or go on about it. Instead, say something like, 'Oh well, if you want to know more about safe drinking limits for older people take a look at these websites', and then drop the subject, for the time being at least.

You could try setting a good example yourself – cut back your own drinking to the safe limits; don't automatically offer your parents a drink when they come to see you, or automatically open a bottle or two of wine with dinner; encourage them to take part in activities and hobbies that don't involve alcohol; experiment with non-alcoholic drinks when you have an evening out.

After all, you're not being a spoilsport or trying to ruin your parents' social life, you're trying to help them have a contented and healthy old age. The occasional drink can be one of life's pleasures, but being an elderly drunk doesn't qualify as fun. One of the older drinkers interviewed for *Panorama* described crawling to the toilet the morning after because he couldn't stand up. Waking up unable to remember how they got home or – even worse – remembering making a complete fool of themselves, or lying in a pool of their own urine, is no way for older people, especially those you love, to spend their later years.

Help for older drinkers

Help does exist, and the GP should be the first port of call once your relative has agreed that there might be a problem. Or he or she could contact one of the organizations dedicated to helping those who need it. The Royal College of Psychiatrists says that actually drink problems are easier to treat in older people than in younger generations. They suggest trying the following.

- A 'detox' programme, which involves giving the person medication to reduce any withdrawal symptoms and gradually reducing the dose after days or weeks.
- Support groups, of which Alcoholics Anonymous is the best known (see Useful addresses). Its famous '12-step' programme can be very successful, but is not for everyone. It may also be difficult for someone with mobility problems to get to AA meetings.
- Talking therapies – the GP should be able to make a referral to a local service.
- A change in routine, so that alcohol becomes a less vital part of life.
- Dealing with the problem that led to the drinking, whether it's loneliness and isolation, or depression, in other, less destructive ways.

5

Dementia

Healthcare professionals and politicians agree that dementia is one of the most important challenges facing today's society. With the increase in life expectancy comes a parallel increase in the number of old and frail people suffering from dementia, which is primarily a condition of extreme old age.

Dementia – or more properly the dementias, as there are several different forms of the illness with different symptoms and treatments – currently affects about 800,000 people in the UK and this is predicted to rise to over a million by 2021. Family carers are currently saving the country more than £8 billion a year by caring for their relatives at home and there are continual debates about the best way for very sick old people to be looked after.

Facts and figures about the extent and cost of dementia care only tell half the story. As anyone who has seen a loved one 'disappear' through the ravages of these distressing conditions knows, dementia can be heartbreaking for both the carer and the cared for. Those caring for someone with dementia suffer a double bereavement – first when the person they once knew and loved becomes an aggressive, confused or unresponsive stranger, and again when that person finally passes away. Caring for a parent with dementia can be challenging and frustrating – though occasionally rewarding, too. You know that it is the illness, and not Mum or Dad, who is telling you to get lost or accusing you of stealing their pension money, who repeats the same questions time after time after time, who hides their false teeth in the fridge and doesn't recognize their once loved granddaughter, but that doesn't make the experience any less harrowing.

What is dementia?

Dementia is a progressive, degenerative disease of the brain, which causes nerve cells to die in particular areas. Symptoms will vary according to the part of the brain that is affected. As yet, research has been unable to discover exactly why this happens. The result is that the nerve cells that transmit messages are disrupted and the person slowly loses the ability to function effectively in the world. Memory loss is just one of the most common symptoms, but some forms of dementia affect different nerve cells and produce different symptoms such as changes in personality and behaviour.

Alzheimer's disease is the best-known and commonest form of dementia, affecting something like 55 per cent of those with the condition. People with Alzheimer's produce less of a vital brain chemical called acetylcholine, which carries messages and instructions between brain cells in the areas of the brain responsible for memory. Fragments of an abnormal substance called beta-amyloid protein are deposited in the damaged areas.

As far as we know, there is no way to prevent the development of Alzheimer's, although there is some evidence that a healthy diet and lifestyle can reduce the risk.

Vascular dementia happens when damage to the blood vessels leads to the brain being deprived of oxygen. Vascular dementia can be stroke-related, with brain damage happening after a stroke or a series of mini-strokes. Depression, mood swings and sometimes epilepsy can result. Another form of vascular dementia is the result of damage to the blood vessels deep inside the brain.

Lewy body dementia, like Alzheimer's, is associated with abnormal protein deposits in nerve cells, causing damage to them. We don't yet know why this happens, but the 'Lewy bodies' are also found in the brains of people with Parkinson's disease, and the effects may be similar – slowness, stiffness and shaking limbs.

Pick's disease, otherwise known as fronto-temporal dementia, can affect younger people and is also characterized by abnormal proteins found in the brain, but they are different proteins and affect different parts of the brain. Pick's disease can produce personality and behavioural changes rather than memory loss, as with Alzheimer's.

Other illnesses that can produce dementia-type symptoms in their later stages include Huntington's, a hereditary disorder of the central nervous system, Creutzfeld-Jakob disease, which came to prominence during the BSE scare of the 1990s, HIV and AIDS, motor neurone disease, multiple sclerosis, Parkinson's disease and long-standing alcohol abuse.

Because there are so many different types of dementia producing so many different symptoms, it can be surprisingly difficult to obtain a definite diagnosis. The Alzheimer's Society says that only 43 per cent of those who have the condition have actually been accurately diagnosed. It is important to remember that there are other conditions that affect older people, such as depression, or an underactive thyroid gland, which can produce very similar symptoms, such as confusion and forgetfulness. The everyday absent-mindedness we're all familiar with, such as forgetting someone's name temporarily, or popping the car keys down somewhere and being totally unable to recall where they are, do not necessarily mean that dementia is on the horizon.

Symptoms to look out for

So what *should* be a cause for concern if you are caring for an elderly and difficult person? And what can you do to help them? Carers often say that the first thing they notice is that the person 'didn't seem quite himself/herself'.

- Look out for an increase in absent-mindedness and more lapses of memory. Dementia often affects short-term memory first. Your relative might be able to chat quite happily about 'the old days' but be unable to recall what they had for breakfast or remember an appointment.
- The person may get tired more easily than before.
- He or she may find it hard to learn anything new.
- Repetitive statements or questions may become noticeable.
- Behaviour that seems odd or unlike the person may become more frequent: for example, losing interest in their appearance when they have always been fastidious, or using unfamiliar bad language.
- Be aware of any sense of disorientation in time and place; perhaps the person will get up for work when it's the weekend or forget a well-known route to the shops.

Getting help

Quite a lot of help is available for people with dementia and their carers. Your first port of call should always be your parent's GP. The first problem you are likely to encounter is a reluctance to make an appointment, as the person may not be aware, or may not want to admit, that there is anything wrong. You may be able to convince them that a 'general check-up' could be a good idea, or persuade them to go to have a chat about another condition they may have, from a chest infection to a hearing problem. Here's Brenda's story.

> I had been worried about my dad for some time as he was becoming extremely forgetful. Mum is diabetic, though, and eventually she and I managed to convince Dad that their GP wanted to see them both for a check-up. We explained about Dad's memory problems and he was referred to our local memory clinic and eventually given Aricept, one of the drugs intended to slow down the progress of dementia. He is doing very well on it and seems a lot brighter and more interested in life.

There isn't, at present, a simple test that a GP can do that will prove that your parent definitely has dementia. Most of the tests and observations that are offered are designed to rule out other possibilities, such as depression or a thyroid disorder. The GP will ask questions about symptoms and also check things like blood pressure and cholesterol levels, as well as finding out whether your parent is a smoker or has diabetes – any of which might mean that they are at higher risk of a stroke or vascular dementia.

Most areas of the UK now have 'memory clinics', where those with symptoms of dementia can be carefully assessed by specialist teams of neurologists, nurses and other experts. A simple test called the MMSE (mini mental state examination) is often applied to assess people's mental condition. This involves asking them a series of simple questions such as the date and the name of the town they live in. They may also be asked to name familiar objects like a watch or a pen, to repeat a sequence of words and copy out a sentence. From the answers given the nurses will offer a treatment plan, which may involve medication if it is required, plus follow-up visits. Counselling and support for carers are part of the treatment offered.

Treatment for dementia

There is no cure for dementia at the present time and it is a degenerative condition, which means that your relative's symptoms will worsen over time, and this is something you need to prepare for. However, research is ongoing and there are grounds for cautious optimism. The 13-year, internationally based human genome project identified all the approximately 25,000 genes in human DNA, and increased scientists' understanding of both genetic disease and key biochemical processes. This enhanced knowledge means that research that might once have taken five years can now be completed in six months.

Having said that there is no cure, there are drug treatments that can help, and also other ways of managing the condition to make life more comfortable and enjoyable for both dementia patients and their carers.

Drug treatments for dementia came on to the market in the late 1990s; although they are not a cure, they can stabilize the symptoms of mild to moderate dementia and prevent them getting any worse, albeit for a limited amount of time. Three drugs known as acetylcholinesterase inhibitors are now available, and one of these may be prescribed to reduce the breakdown of the brain chemical acetylcholine, which, as we have seen, is what happens in Alzheimer's disease.

These three drugs – donepezil (brand name Aricept), rivastigmine (brand name Exelon) and galantamine (brand name Reminyl) – have been recommended for use in cases of mild to moderate dementia since October 2010. They may help with the commonest symptoms, such as memory loss and confusion. Which drug the doctors prescribe will depend on the person's symptoms, any side effects that develop, and the type of dementia diagnosed or suspected.

A fourth drug, memantine (brand name Ebixa), is now available to treat moderate to severe dementia. It works in a slightly different way from the others and has been used in combination with Aricept in the USA with some success.

Existing drugs, such as tranquillizers, can also be prescribed to treat some of the most distressing symptoms of dementia, such as aggression or anxiety. Until very recently anti-psychotics were used in this way, but dementia care experts now feel that more effective ways of 'managing' difficult behaviour can mean a better quality of life for people with dementia and those caring for them.

Caring for someone with dementia

Dementia produces different symptoms in different people. It's a condition that is as individual as the people who have it. It changes some people's personalities and exaggerates qualities that have always been present in others. This means that day-to-day management is different for everyone. Some people, even those living alone, manage quite well with just a little help. It may be that they are experiencing nothing more than what is known as 'minor cognitive impairment' which could mean vagueness, forgetfulness and confusion.

The effect on other people can be very much harder to deal with. They can become aggressive, nervous, bewildered, argumentative and generally difficult to care for. Things that sound like minor symptoms, such as repeating the same questions over and over, or following you around, or forgetting how to dress or brush their hair or teeth, can try the patience of even the most well-meaning carer.

The most important thing to remember is that *it's the illness that is causing all these problems*. Your mum or dad is not behaving in this way to annoy you. He or she really can't help it – and the chances are that your parent feels more scared, frustrated and unhappy than you do.

Knowing all that doesn't stop you finding the things they do exasperating, but it does help you to develop reserves of patience. Perhaps take a deep breath and go into another room to cool down rather than snap at Mum when she asks you for the umpteenth time where Granddad is – when Granddad actually passed away 30 years ago.

What seems like difficult behaviour – refusing to eat, or go to bed – is often people's coded way of communicating. What you, as carer, have to try to do is work out what they are really trying to tell you. Remember that to someone with dementia the world seems like a frightening place and nothing makes sense any more. They may be in pain, hungry, thirsty, or need the loo. They may be refusing to cooperate for various reasons:

- They don't understand what they are being asked to do.
- They feel they are being patronized or 'bossed about' when they want to remain in control.
- They don't know why they need help with personal care, such as having a bath or using the toilet.
- If they refuse to eat, this may be because they don't like what is served, they have forgotten how to use a knife and fork – or they may have toothache or problems with their dentures!
- They have forgotten what their medication is for.

It can help if you let your parent continue with familiar routines as far as possible. Familiarity can be soothing even in a world that has stopped making sense. If Dad has always preferred a strip-wash to a modern shower, let him carry on doing it his way. If Mum always liked to be up, dressed and with her hair done before she had breakfast, keep up the habit.

So just how *do* you deal with difficult behaviour in people with dementia? Health professionals point out that the two key things to try are distraction and reassurance.

Distraction might perhaps consist of putting on some familiar music, offering a magazine to look at, or going for a walk; sometimes simply sitting by the window watching passers-by can also be comforting.

Reassurance is important too. If your parent doesn't always remember who you are – or who anyone is – gently remind them rather than getting upset yourself. Leave that for later. If they seem unhappy or agitated, remind them that everything is all right and you are taking care of things.

The Alzheimer's Society (see Useful addresses) offers useful tips on communicating with those who have dementia. This is its advice.

- Listen carefully to what they have to say.
- Make sure you have their full attention before you speak. Don't stand over them, as this can seem intimidating.
- Pay attention to their body language.
- Speak clearly.
- Think about how things appear to them.
- Use physical contact to reassure them.
- Show respect and patience, remembering that it may take longer for their brain to process the information you are giving them, and to respond.
- Let them express their feelings. Sometimes it's best just to listen and show you care.

The Society runs online forums for those with dementia and their carers and you will find lots of helpful tips and hints on coping with challenging behaviour. Whether your parent has become aggressive, wanders at night or in the daytime, shouts and screams, hides and loses possessions, accuses you or someone else of stealing, attacking or molesting them, has become incontinent or started to display inappropriate sexual behaviour, there will be other carers who have dealt with the same issues. You are not alone.

Practical help

There are practical ways in which you can help those who are only mildly affected by dementia, who are still able to run their own lives with minimal support. Diaries, pinboards and Post-It notes can be used to remind forgetful older folk that they go to the day centre on Wednesdays, and the community nurse comes round on Fridays.

We have already mentioned the importance of a regular, familiar routine. Make sure that everyday objects are always kept in the same place – keys on the same hook, glasses next to the sofa, coffee mugs next to the kettle. As the disease progresses it may be helpful to put labels on the doors saying 'kitchen' or 'bathroom' – or even a picture of the cooker and fridge or the toilet. Any new information you have to give should be kept simple and repeated as often as necessary: 'We're going to the clinic tomorrow', or 'It's time for your pills now'. Give them time to take in what you have said and pay attention to the way you say things. Calmness reassures; a loud voice and agitation on your part will only frighten your parent and won't help them to understand what is required of them.

Everyday tasks can be broken down into small, manageable steps and it's helpful to let the person do as much as he can for himself, rather than 'taking over'. Try to do things *with* your relative, rather than *for* him. Encourage him to carry on with simple household tasks where possible and to continue with hobbies and interests. Exercise can be useful too – just because his memory is going, it doesn't mean that he doesn't need to get out and about and keep as fit as possible. This also has the benefit of tiring the person out so he is less likely to wake up in the night and wander.

On the other hand, too much hustle and bustle and too many changes of scene can be worrying for the person with dementia. You need to be guided by his needs and moods and allow him to concentrate on one thing at a time.

It is obviously very important that your parent is safe, whether they are still able to live independently or are living with you. Make sure that common-sense safety precautions are in place, such as good lighting, non-slip rugs, handrails on the stairs and the bath, and smoke alarms. You may need to fit locks on doors and some cupboards if your parent is inclined to wander, or hide things.

It's also sensible to alert local people – the neighbours, the corner shop, even the police – and let them know that your relative has memory problems, so that she can be escorted home if she gets lost.

Assistive technology

Sometimes known as 'telecare', modern technology can be extremely useful in helping older people with memory problems to retain some independence. It can also be very reassuring for their family and carers. Most of us will be familiar with simple versions, such as smoke alarms and the buttons and pull-cords seen in sheltered housing and disabled toilets, which enable people to call for help if needed.

The Social Services in many areas offer 'community alarm' systems, often in the form of pendants or wristlets, which can be worn by frail older people to call for help if they have a fall. There are also much more sophisticated aids and sensors that remind people to take their medication regularly, or raise the alarm if someone falls out of bed, wets the bed, leaves the gas on or taps running, or tries to leave the house during the night. Telecare systems like this are linked via the phone line to a monitoring service that either reassures the person that everything is fine, or alerts named carers, family or the emergency services.

There are special vibrating alarms for those who are hard of hearing, and 'location sensors' (similar to satnavs) which enable those who wander off and get lost to be found again.

You can find out more about the assistive technology available either from your local Social Services department or from the Disabled Living Foundation (see Useful addresses). Once you begin to feel that your parent can no longer manage independently or with occasional help from the family, you should apply for a care assessment from the Social Services. We will look at how best to do this in Chapter 8.

Who else can help?

We have already mentioned memory clinics, which are staffed by experts in the diagnosis and treatment of dementia. You will also come into contact with community psychiatric nurses (CPNs), who are there to offer help and advice, not only to the person with dementia but to carers as well.

Their job is to visit as often as necessary to help assess your parent's ability to cope with 'activities of daily living', which can cover anything from shopping and cooking to handling finances, in the early stages of the illness, right through to appropriate care when dementia has become more advanced. They have wide experience in dealing with challenging behaviour and may be able to offer helpful solutions, as well as being a 'listening ear' for carers.

The staff at the memory clinic and the CPN will be able to tell you if there are day centres that offer respite care, so that you, the carer, can have a break – and also how to persuade your parent that going to a day centre is a good idea! Local carers' groups and support groups run by the Alzheimer's Society can also offer a lifeline. If your parent has another kind of dementia, for instance Pick's disease or Huntington's, there are specialist support groups who can help.

Most people have heard of Macmillan nurses who specialize in the care of cancer patients and their families. Fewer know about Admiral nurses, who perform a similar function for those with dementia and their carers. There may be an Admiral nurse in your area, or you can call their national helpline (see Useful addresses).

The charity Vitalise organizes holidays for disabled people in several centres around the UK, and runs special weeks for those with dementia and their carers (see Useful addresses).

About a third of the people who have Alzheimer's disease are in residential care, according to the Alzheimer's Society. The time will eventually come when you have to begin to think about this option for your parent, and we will look at the best way to make this choice in the next chapter.

6

When to step in and offer help

Watching a much-loved parent – or even one who has always been difficult and demanding – become more and more frail can never be easy. Although we all know, logically, that our parents are growing older and may need our help one day, it can still be a shock when it happens. Just how do you decide that Mum and Dad aren't coping and perhaps shouldn't be living on their own? How do you tell them, tactfully, that help is needed? And, last but not least, is there any way of persuading stubborn and independent older people that help is there to be claimed and should be accepted?

Do they really need help?

If you ask whether they are all right, the chances are that your parents will say they are. We have already seen in Chapter 2 that it's hard for people to admit that they can no longer manage to do things they once took for granted. They may genuinely feel that everything is fine, or may be reluctant to admit to their families that that isn't the case. It may be the result of pride or reluctance to worry you.

Many old people are really afraid of 'being put into a home', for reasons that are perfectly understandable. They don't want to give up the home they may have lived in for 40 years. They don't want to give up their independence or feel that they have to rely on other people to make their meals, tell them when to get up and go to bed, when to bath or use the toilet. 'Old people's homes' don't have a good image, even though many are excellent and can be the best option for very frail, sick people or those with advanced dementia.

However, if your parents aren't in that position, but are just finding it hard to cope with their present living conditions, there are lots of other options.

It's vital to remember that any decisions about their future must be taken *by all of you* – not by you on behalf of your parents, unless they are absolutely unable to do so. There should be no question of them being 'put' in a home, or anywhere else. They still have rights, even the right to refuse help.

If you live near your parents and see them regularly, you might not notice their increasing frailty. If you live miles away and only come to visit a few times a year, you might be shocked at the changes you see. Offering help isn't a question of imposing your standards on them. They don't have to have the latest kitchen equipment, a flat-screen TV and a superfast broadband connection – but they *do* need to be warm, clean and well fed. It's when it seems that these basic needs are not being met that the warning bells should start to ring.

Signs to look out for include:

- weight loss;
- bruising on arms or legs – this could be the result of frequent falls;
- a grubby or untidy kitchen – burned pans could indicate that they are forgetting to turn the cooker off;
- bills piling up and threats to cut off the gas/electricity – if this is happening, make sure the energy company knows they are dealing with vulnerable older people;
- little food in the fridge, or food that is past its sell-by date;
- increasing forgetfulness – frequently losing keys or glasses, getting lost in familiar places;
- untidy or unkempt appearance – signs of self-neglect;
- loss of interest in family, friends or hobbies.

Consultant clinical psychologist Dr Pat Frankish says that if you do begin to feel that Mum and Dad are not really coping any longer, the most tactful approach is to begin to help quietly, without making too much of it.

For example, you might visit more often, and take a pie prepared for them with a comment like, 'I was making one for us and I thought you might like one too.' Then you might offer to pop to the shops or mow the lawn. Elderly people will often say yes if they think they are making *you* feel better.

Sometimes it helps to say you have heard about attendance allowance and offer to help them make a claim. It is possible that the prospect of more funds might be a motivator. If there is a sibling group, it can be helpful for one to visit and tell them that you have all had a discussion and would feel better if you would let *x* or *y* happen (perhaps getting a weekly cleaner, or some grab rails in the bathroom). Sometimes everyone agreeing makes it easier.

There will be individual differences. The key factor is to help your parents to keep their independence as long as possible, but to make sure they know that you want to help and would feel bad if they, for example, had a fall because they weren't getting the help they need.

Persuading your parents that change is needed

This can be a struggle! Remember that they are dealing with loss – of their physical and mental skills, their independence, their privacy, and this is bound to be hard for them. We have already seen that they may be feeling frightened, angry, or guilty about 'being a burden', and afraid to admit that they can't manage as they are any longer. When you are discussing changes, choose a time when all of you are relaxed, and ask *them* what *they* think. You can't impose solutions on your parents, and if they feel that they are being railroaded into making a choice that is not their own, they could dig their heels in.

Probably the most common scenario is that your parents are living in a house that no longer meets their needs. It may be too big, too cold, too isolated, too inconvenient or a combination of all of those things. However, it is also their home. They may have lived there for 30, 40 or 50 years, and the idea of moving out may be upsetting, from both a practical and an emotional point of view.

A house move is not the only option. There is an enormous range of practical aids for elderly, frail and disabled people, and there are also thousands of pounds in unclaimed benefits for them – we investigate these in Chapter 8. The first possibility to consider is arranging for your parents to remain where they are – if this is what they want – by adapting their home to make it more suitable for them.

Staying put

Age UK have an extremely useful booklet called 'Adapting Your Home', containing details of all the help that is available to enable older people to stay in their own homes for as long as possible. You'll need to work out exactly what it is that they find difficult or impossible at the moment. For instance, if they can no longer manage stairs easily and they only have an upstairs bathroom and toilet, possibilities may include installing a stairlift, or putting in a downstairs bathroom, shower and/or toilet; the loan of a commode might also be a temporary solution.

For major works of this kind, the best way to begin is by calling the Social Services and asking for a 'care assessment' (more about what is involved in this on p. 62). Many people do not realize that all community equipment and adaptations that cost less than £1,000 are provided and fitted free of charge and regardless of means – in England at least. (The rules in Scotland are slightly different.) This can cover things like grab rails in the bath or shower, lever taps, which older people find easier to use, or a short ramp to help your parents get into and out of their home.

For any adaptations that cost more than £1,000 – for instance, an additional ground-floor room that is wheelchair accessible – it is necessary to apply for funding in the form of a disabled facilities grant. Again, the Social Services can give you information about this. Homeowners and tenants can apply and the DFG is means-tested.

If your parents are council or housing association tenants, the local Housing Office should be able to inform them about adapting their home. Homeowners or private tenants should contact a home improvement agency (sometimes known as Care and Repair, or Staying Put). These are not-for-profit organizations that help older people to adapt their homes and can also give information about disabled facilities grants.

Both Age UK (and other charities such as the Royal British Legion) and some councils run 'handyperson schemes' to help older people with small household repairs.

If your parents are no longer interested in cooking for themselves, or are not able to, the Royal Voluntary Service (formerly known as WRVS) can provide Meals on Wheels, or companies such as Wiltshire Farm Foods will deliver healthy, nutritionally balanced meals, which are stored in the freezer and then heated up in a microwave.

Many people will be familiar with the Careline schemes run by local councils, where a pendant or wristband is provided for older people so that they can call for help if, for example, they have a fall and are unable to reach a phone. Telecare, or assistive technology (see p. 39), is now much more sophisticated than that, and enables older people who are frail or even in the early stages of dementia to continue to live at home. For information about this, again, the Social Services should be your first port of call.

We will look at how to get a care assessment from the Social Services in Chapter 8, but of course there is no reason why you can't explore the possibility of employing a private carer at any stage. Contact the UK Homecare Association (see Useful addresses) for more information about home care.

If your parents don't need much help, just someone to look in on them regularly and let you know how they are, a trusted neighbour might be willing to do this. If your parents have a religious faith you could approach their local church, mosque or synagogue. Befriending services with local volunteers are offered by charities such as Age UK, the Royal Voluntary Service, the British Red Cross and the Salvation Army.

Gentle persuasion

The best way to get your parents to agree to be helped is by gentle persuasion, always remembering that, in the end, it is their choice. Take it slowly, one step at a time. You might suggest that a once-a-week cleaning lady would save them having to do 'the rough work', and that bath aids or handrails would enable Mum to enjoy a warm bath again without having to worry about slipping and falling, or being unable to get out. Suggest, don't insist – and give them time to think about whether whatever you're suggesting would be a good idea.

You could try telling Mum that you think Dad needs a bit of help, and vice versa. You could say that you know you're silly to worry about them, but you do . . . and that you'd feel so much happier if you knew that they could call for help if they had a fall, or whatever your suggestion was.

Always present any changes as positive steps that will maintain or even increase their independence, rather than making it sound as if they are too old and feeble to manage alone. For instance, using a wheelchair would mean Dad could still enjoy his outings rather than being confined to the house. Having ready-prepared meals delivered means that Mum wouldn't have to be bothered cooking. Employing a cleaner would mean fewer chores to do, as well as some company.

Enrol some allies if your parents still seem unsure or reluctant. Do they have friends who use wheelchairs or mobility scooters, who have their meals delivered or go to a local day centre? Would they be more likely to listen to the doctor, or a contemporary (or a contemporary who *was* a doctor)? Or a minister of religion or someone else they respect?

Moving in with family

Sometimes, this is a happy solution for everyone. Families, after all, are there to look after one another through good times and bad, and in some cultures it's unthinkable for older family members to live anywhere other than with their sons and daughters. However, it isn't the right answer for everyone and needs to be carefully thought through. There are many questions to ask yourselves.

- Which family member will Mum or Dad live with, and how will the others feel?
- Is the family member likely to move house (for work reasons, perhaps) in the next few years, and how might this affect Mum or Dad?
- Is the house really big enough for an extra person to move in and be comfortable?
- Are there financial considerations? Does Mum or Dad have a property to sell? How will this affect the siblings? Will your parent pay rent or contribute to household bills? Will the family home have to be adapted to make it suitable for a frail older person, and if it does, who will pay for this?
- How do the grandchildren feel about it?
- What sort of support services are available for older people in the area?
- What other commitments do the family have – to work, children, grandchildren? How will this fit in with new caring responsibilities?

Plus, of course, you should consider how your parents feel about the move themselves! If they are country-lovers, could they cope with a move to the town or city – or vice versa? Would they be leaving a circle of friends and acquaintances behind and be worried about making friends in a new area? How would they feel about sharing a home with boisterous children or noisy teenagers, even if they love them dearly?

Here's Sarah's story.

Dad has been an invalid for many years – he had a stroke which left him with speech and mobility problems. Mum was his carer, but then she had a heart attack and died very suddenly. We never really thought of Dad going into residential care; it was understood that he would come to us.

We have an extra downstairs room, which we turned into a bed-sitter for him so he could have his own furniture and TV. I thought I could just go to work in the morning and pop back at lunch time to see him. I soon realized that he really couldn't manage to get himself dressed and make breakfast, so I gave up my job to become his full-time carer. He doesn't need nursing, just someone with him most of the time.

I'm used to it now, but if I'm honest I have to admit it has been a struggle. Basically, I was bored to death and Dad was, too. I have now found a place for him in a day centre he goes to twice a week. He enjoys the company and it gives me a bit of freedom. My husband is a tower of strength but we have three teenagers and it's hard for them. I used to spend half my time saying 'Sssh!' to them, but I realized that it's their home too and if Dad finds their music and computer games annoying, he has to learn to give and take as well.

We have a fortnight's respite care so we can go away on holiday, which is wonderful. I know my sister feels guilty that she's not able to help more, but her house doesn't even have a downstairs loo so even a visit is a problem. We just take it all a day at a time. I sometimes wonder that if we had thought it through we might have made a different choice – for Dad's sake as well as ours.

Retirement housing

Retirement housing, sometimes known as sheltered housing, is a good option for older folk who want to retain their independence but need the reassurance of knowing that help is available if it's needed. Sheltered flats or bungalows have their own front doors and are planned to be suitable for older people with lifts to upper floors, grab rails and non-slip flooring, as well as alarm cords or buttons in each room. There is normally a manager on-site, who can't offer personal or nursing care but who acts as a 'good neighbour'. Other facilities vary but most have communal lounges and gardens, laundry rooms and guest suites for visitors. Social activities are often arranged by the residents, but of course these are entirely optional.

Retirement housing can be bought or rented. Most flats are sold on a leasehold basis and there is a service charge. You'll need to check exactly what this covers and whether it is likely to increase.

Some councils offer financial incentives to older tenants who want to downsize, freeing up a family home in the process. Most sheltered housing schemes are conveniently situated near to local shops and facilities like doctors' surgeries and the post office. Some are in the form of 'retirement villages' where there is a care home to which residents can move as they become more frail. Those living in sheltered flats are entitled to exactly the same care services from the local council as they are in other types of accommodation.

Other types of sheltered housing, sometimes known as 'extra care' or 'very sheltered' housing, are suitable for those who need a little more support – for example, if your parents need meals prepared for them. Abbeyfield houses come into this category. Residents have their own rooms with private facilities, and two main meals prepared for them every day. Abbeyfield houses don't, however, provide personal or nursing care. Charities such as Age UK and the Elderly Accommodation Counsel can provide more information about retirement housing (for contact details of these organizations, see Useful addresses).

Care homes

There may come a time when residential care really is the best option for your parent or parents. They may have become extremely frail, sick, or be suffering from advanced dementia so that they are unable to live at home any longer, even with support from family and the Social Services. They may need personal care – help with dressing, bathing, eating and drinking, using the toilet, moving around – or nursing care such as changing dressings, or administering medication.

Families often feel that they have failed when a parent has to go into full-time care, but this really isn't so. The best care homes offer not only day-to-day care but also company and activities that residents can enjoy as far as they are able – anything from art classes to regular outings, which families simply couldn't provide at home. Here's Lorna's story.

Mum was in a sheltered flat in a London suburb and we live two hours' drive away. She is blind and has severe arthritis and the manager kept calling us to tell us she really didn't think Mum could manage on her own any longer. Mum always said that she wanted to die in her own home, so of course that was what we wanted for her too, but we became aware that she needed nursing care. Being blind, she wasn't really comfortable in my house, and I couldn't lift her when she needed help.

I knew nothing about care homes, except the horror stories you see in the press and on TV! I contacted the council, the CAB and Age UK, who were very helpful. I went to see lots of homes I wasn't happy with but then found a lovely one, just five miles from my house. It's a converted manor house so doesn't feel like an 'institution' and the staff are warm and kind. Both Mum and I liked it at once.

She has her own room with her own furniture and a bell she can ring, day or night, if she needs help. She has breakfast and tea in her room and lunch in the dining room with the other residents, some of whom have become her friends. She goes to a local Blind Club and there are outings. Being so near, I can see her almost every day, my brother and the grandchildren visit, and if there are any worries I can always talk them over with the staff. I think we have found the best solution for all of us.

While political arguments rage about how, exactly, care for very old and frail people should be funded, it is still down to families to find suitable care for their elderly parents. Age UK is a fabulous resource for this as they update their information regularly. The rules on care are complex and are changing all the time. Old people's homes used to be either 'residential' or 'nursing'. The latter were required to have qualified nursing staff available at all times. Currently, care homes may be described as 'with nursing care' or 'with dementia care', so you need to look for somewhere offering an appropriate level of care for your parent. The Alzheimer's Society can offer advice on the best care homes for dementia patients.

The Age UK website has a checklist describing what you should look for in a care home. Most will send out a brochure describing what they offer residents, but there's no substitute for a visit. This will be your parent's home. As well as being scrupulously clean, warm and comfortable, you'll need to consider factors like:

- how near it is for family visits and how welcome visitors are;
- whether residents can bring their own furniture, belongings, pets;
- what activities are provided for residents;
- what meals are provided and whether special dietary requirements are catered for;
- whether residents can make their own drinks and snacks if required;
- whether residents' privacy is respected;
- whether there is access to a garden.

Talk to the manager, the staff, and other residents and their families, and that will give you an idea of the way the home is run. Take your time; it's a big decision. Some homes offer prospective residents the opportunity to spend some time – a weekend, perhaps, or a longer period of respite care – with them to see if they like it. This could be a good way of 'easing in' a parent who is doubtful or reluctant to move.

The question of who pays for care of the elderly is a complex one. How much any individual pays will depend on their personal circumstances, and also on where they live. Nursing care is free in England, but personal care has to be paid for. In Scotland both are free. Financial help is often available with care home fees. BUPA, which runs private care homes, says about half of their residents receive help with the fees.

Residents are expected to claim any benefits to put towards care home fees. Exactly how much is charged depends on your parents' income, including pensions and savings. They will not have to sell their home to pay for their care if it is lived in by their wife, husband, partner, a relative aged under 16 or over 60, or a disabled relative under 60.

Even if you can afford to, and plan to, pay for care privately, it's best to obtain a Social Services assessment (see p. 62) for your parent, in case their circumstances change.

Moving out

Once you have persuaded Mum and Dad that the move is necessary, don't underestimate the physical and emotional demands the actual move will make. A house move is an upheaval for anyone, especially for those who are old and in indifferent health, who may have lived in their present home for more than 40 years.

Encourage your parents to start clearing their home well in advance. A lifetime of assorted clutter takes a lot of shifting. Enlist the help of family and friends and let your parents supervise and decide which of their belongings are going with them. Some can be left as part of the fixtures and fittings in their old home, some can be passed on to friends and relatives, some will go to the local charity shop and some to the council recycling centre. Be prepared for arguments – but also for some nostalgic moments as you unearth old treasures from the attic or the garden shed.

Some removal companies specialize in moving older people, such as Seamless Relocation (<www.seamlessrelocation.com>) – or you could ask locally for recommendations.

7

Helping to improve the quality of life

Have you ever thought that one reason why your parents might be hard work is simply because they are bored? Social isolation and loneliness, whether or not they are accompanied by poor health and physical frailty, can make people behave in ways that seem demanding to those who are trying to care for them.

Company and interests

The stereotype of the 'lonely old person' does have its roots in reality. According to a poll carried out by the Scottish Widows finance company in December 2011, almost half of over-sixties live on their own. Among those over 75, half see family members less than once a month and only a quarter have weekly visits from family. There is evidence that isolation is bad for people. A huge research study in the USA, involving more than 300,000 people over seven years, found that those with 'strong social relationships' had a 50 per cent increased likelihood of survival compared with those leading solitary lives. As long ago as 1988, *Science* magazine was suggesting that loneliness was a health risk analogous to smoking, high blood pressure, lack of exercise and obesity. Age UK say that half of older people consider the television their main source of company.

Before you rush round and enrol your parent in the local day centre, though, do bear in mind that not everyone wants to be surrounded by other people all the time. Plenty of older folk are perfectly happy with their own company. It's all about person-centred care, remember? That means knowing your parent or parents well enough to suggest activities that they will actually enjoy. Here's Marcia, aged 79.

My local church organizes a 'Friendship Day' every few months for local older people. They mean well and put a lot of work into it and I've been a couple of times, but too many assumptions are made about what 'old people' want to do or like doing. For instance, they organize a sing-song around the piano. I'm tone-deaf, always have been, and find the idea of singing in public excruciatingly embarrassing. I don't like Bingo either, and am not at all craft-minded, so knitting and craftwork are not for me. I appreciate the company and I'm sure the organizers think I'm a miserable old bat, but we don't all enjoy the same things just because we're old, any more than younger people do!

Marcia has a point. Not all the activities available to older people in their area will appeal to your parents. However, it's a good idea to find out what *is* available and then suggest that they might like to try one or more of them. Explain that they're not signing up for life, and if the day centre or lunch club turns out not to be their sort of thing, there are plenty more activities to try.

You can find out from the council, your local paper, or Age UK what sort of events and activities are organized locally for older folk. Churches and community centres are other sources of information. Day centres and lunch clubs specifically for older people often provide a hot lunch as well as company and activities.

Shared interest groups are not necessarily restricted to older people. Your parent might enjoy a reading group, a local history group, a photography club, a choir, amateur dramatics – the possibilities are endless.

Support groups for people with particular disabilities, or their carers, can be a chance to let off steam. It can be very therapeutic to spend time with others who know exactly what your problems are because they share them. If your parent has sight or hearing problems, mobility issues, is a cancer survivor, has been bereaved or has Alzheimer's, the relevant charity will be able to provide details of local support.

Many organizations have befrienders who are keen to visit and have friendly relationships with isolated older people. Both parties gain from this and those involved always say that it's as much fun for the visitor as the visited if they really hit it off! The Royal Voluntary Service, the British Red Cross and the Salvation Army are among the charities who do this. There is also Contact the Elderly, which organizes monthly tea parties in members' homes for older people (for contact details of all these organizations, see Useful addresses).

As mentioned in Chapter 2, the Internet is a fantastic resource for anyone who is restricted by mobility problems or even housebound. The World Wide Web is exactly that – worldwide. Not only does it make it possible for your parents to research their family tree, or see photographs of the street where they were born, they can make contact with old friends via social networking, or make new ones who share their passion for steam trains, MGM musicals or the adventures of Billy Bunter as described by Frank Richards! There are online discussion groups for literally every kind of interest you – or your parents – can possibly think of, and lots that will never even have crossed your minds.

Another possibility your parents might consider, if they are still living in a larger family home, is renting out one or more rooms. Local colleges and universities are often looking for suitable accommodation for both staff and students. As well as young company, your parents could make up to £4,250 per year in tax-free income through a government scheme called Rent a Room – see <www.direct.gov.uk> for details.

Work and skills

Older people, we know, don't want to be 'written off' as if they no longer have anything to contribute to the world around them. That is far from the case, whether they are contemplating taking a voluntary job, or simply being there to offer a friendly 'listening ear' for their grandchildren. Lots of people look forward to, and welcome, their retirement but it is a huge lifestyle change that shouldn't be underestimated. There are reasons why some people aged over 65 (and Lottery winners) go on working, and they are not all financial ones. People like to feel that they are contributing and not being 'put out to grass' or 'dumped on the scrapheap'. Newly retired people miss having a reason to get up in the morning, and once the novelty of being able to have a lie-in on a weekday wears off, they can sometimes think, 'Now what?'

According to the Royal Voluntary Service, almost a third of people between 65 and 74, and a fifth of those aged 75 plus, actually do a formal, voluntary job. One organization, the Retired and Senior Volunteer Programme (see Useful addresses), is actively looking for volunteers aged over 80. They say that they want older people to be able to use their life experience to help their local community.

Having a job to go to, even if it's only one day a week, has huge advantages. It gives the day a structure, it offers the opportunity to learn new skills as well as sharing existing skills with other – often younger – people. There is often 'mentoring' work and it can be any-thing from knitting to walking groups.

An older person (perhaps a former teacher?) could volunteer in a school, perhaps listening to youngsters reading, or talking about their own childhood in a Living History project, for instance if they were a Second World War evacuee. Country areas with limited public trans-port often need volunteer drivers to take people to hospital appoint-ments. The Royal Voluntary Service, St John Ambulance, British Red Cross, the National Trust and Samaritans all welcome older volunteers with life experience.

Local campaigns against hospital closures and in favour of com-munity libraries also welcome volunteers, of any age. Charity shops need staff to serve behind the counter or sort and price up donations. Animal rescue centres are always looking for foster carers for aban-doned and mistreated pets, especially older ones who are harder to rehome than lively young puppies and kittens.

Don't underestimate the value of pet ownership to older people, especially those on their own. A charity called the Cinnamon Trust specializes in 'matching up' bereaved pet owners with bereaved ani-mals, to the benefit of both (see Useful addresses).

June, 82, has adopted a series of 'golden oldies' from her local Cats Protection branch:

> I've always loved cats but decided I couldn't cope with kittens climbing up the curtains at my age. My CP 'oldies' have always settled in beauti-fully. Currently I have Mortimer, who must be at least 17. He was in a dreadful state when he was taken to Cats Protection but he's a lovely old boy now and such a soothing companion. Of course it's sad when you lose them, but I have the consolation of knowing I've given all my cats a really happy retirement.

If your parents are in sheltered housing or a care home where pets are not allowed, Pets as Therapy and some rescue organizations run therapy visits from friendly cats and dogs.

Learning in later life

There's absolutely nothing to stop your parents joining a local even-ing class, and it's a popular option for older people. Age UK says that almost three-quarters of older people try new activities after retire-ment, with learning a foreign language being a popular choice.

In 2012 the University of the Third Age celebrated its thirtieth birthday. U3A groups are self-help, self-managed lifelong learning cooperatives for older people. The idea is that those who join are not learning in order to acquire qualifications, but just for fun! Courses can be 'real life' or online, all abilities are catered for, and it's possible to study everything from art to zoology. Because local groups are self-managed, literally any subject can be studied; physical activities might also be on offer, and games like bridge and chess, as well as more academic disciplines.

Diet and exercise

Everyone, whatever their age, feels better if they are healthy and well nourished. Diet – and that doesn't mean slimming – and fitness are just as important for older people as they are for the young, if not more so. A healthy, well-balanced diet and an appropriate fitness regime will make your parents feel and look better. Much is known about the effect of diet on mood, and exercise is sometimes prescribed to help lift mild depression, as we have seen in Chapter 3.

Older people often find that their appetite declines, probably because they are less active than they once were. If your parents are eating smaller meals, it's especially important that what they eat is nourishing. A common complaint is that 'expert advice' changes all the time, often so quickly that it's hard to keep up. It is often worth explaining that in the days when much of the population was genuinely undernourished, higher-fat foods like full-cream milk *were* often recommended. These days, as we all know, obesity is much more of a problem. A healthy, balanced diet for older people, as recommended by the NHS, should consist of the following foods:

- At least five portions a day of vegetables and fruit – as juice, fresh or frozen, added to salads and sandwiches or served with a main meal. The vitamins, minerals and fibre in fruit and veg are good for the immune system.
- Starchy foods like bread, potatoes, rice, noodles and chapattis should make up a third of the diet. Wholewheat and wholemeal versions are particularly good for the digestive system.
- Meat, fish and eggs are needed as sources of protein. It's best to use lean cuts and grill rather than fry. A healthy diet does contain *some*

fats, with the omega-3 fats contained in oily fish beneficial for heart health.
- Milk and dairy products are rich in calcium for bone health. Choose lower-fat versions when you can.

Current advice is to keep high-fat and sugary foods like cakes and biscuits as treats, not to add salt to food to prevent high blood pressure, and sip plenty of water to prevent dehydration. If your parents are fans of health supplements, make sure they check with their GP that these don't interact with any medication they may be on.

It's also very important that your parents keep moving, as much as they can. 'Use it or lose it' is the motto here. If they have always enjoyed a game of tennis or judo or bowls, why give up? As little as 30 minutes a day of walking protects the heart and reduces blood pressure. Exercise can also reduce the risk of diabetes, strokes and some cancers, strengthens bones to help prevent falls and is thought to reduce the risk of, and slow the progress of, dementia.

The trick with exercise, if they haven't been used to it, is to start slowly – and have a check-up with the GP if they are absolute beginners. After that, walking is a good way to start – it's free, it's fun, it can be sociable and you can do it anywhere. Two and a half hours of brisk walking every week (or another 'moderate intensity activity' like dancing, cycling, tennis or keep fit), combined with muscle-strengthening activity such as carrying heavy shopping, digging the garden, push-ups or sit-ups, on two days a week are the recommended levels of activity for those over 65.

As with younger people, the secret is to find a form of exercise they enjoy, so that your parents look forward to their walk round the Botanical Gardens or along the sea front, rather than seeing it as a chore. Local gyms and council leisure centres often run classes in keep fit, yoga, Pilates or t'ai chi especially tailored for older exercisers, and there are 'green gyms' and 'senior playgrounds' with exercise machines in the open air in some areas. Swimming and dancing are other possibilities.

The truth is that you are never too old to keep fit – and if your parents don't believe it, tell them about 101-year-old marathon runner and Olympic torch-bearer Fauja Singh from Ilford, who ran the London Marathon for the last time in 2012 and announced his intention of 'only' running in 5 km and 10 km races after that. He was a comparatively youthful 86 when he started running.

Holidays and travel

If your parents have mobility problems or other health issues, the idea of travelling or booking a holiday can seem daunting. However, a lot has been done to make the business of travel a great deal easier for older and disabled people so that they don't have to give up the idea of 'going places'.

Most people know about the bus pass provided to older people by their local council, which allows free bus travel all over the UK outside peak hours. The London Freedom Pass is especially generous, as holders can travel at any time on the Underground and local train services as well. The rules vary from place to place, as do eligibility criteria. If your parents were born after 5 April 1950, the age at which they can claim their bus pass is changing along with the rise in the pension age. Check with your local council for details.

If they are fans of long-distance coach travel, National Express has a Senior and a Disabled Coachcard, offering one-third off ordinary fares. Train companies have Senior and Disabled Railcards on the same principle. Visually impaired travellers can get a free ticket for a companion. If mobility is a problem or your parents are wheelchair users, the train companies have assisted travel teams – people who can help passengers to get on and off the train as well as assisting with their luggage. Some train stations have lifts for the use of disabled passengers and wheelchairs that can be borrowed for getting around the station. Most ask for 24 hours' notice to provide this help but will do their best to offer assistance at any time. Many buses are now wheelchair accessible, as are London taxis; provision varies in other cities.

Contact your council for details of local accessible transport. Some areas have Dial-a-Ride, wheelchair-accessible minibuses that can be booked like a taxi. If your parents are still able to drive but can't walk far from the car, ask the council about the Blue Badge scheme, which allows people with walking difficulties to park free on yellow lines and in pay and display bays. There are even schemes that help drivers with disabilities to adapt their own cars. Contact the Forum of Mobility Centres (see Useful addresses) for details of this.

Much progress has been made in making tourist attractions, hotels and B&Bs accessible to people with mobility issues, and all local tourist boards will provide information about exactly where visitors with disabilities can and cannot go.

There's really no reason to let frailty or disability hold your parents back if they still want to travel. Some older people become stressed if they are not sure where the nearest toilets are, or whether they will be able to use them. RADAR operate a National Key Scheme, which gives access to more than 9,000 accessible toilets all over the UK. The scheme is administered by Disability Rights UK (see Useful addresses).

Foreign travel is perfectly possible too. Airlines and airports will help passengers with special needs – although, as with train and bus companies, it's important to request help well in advance of the trip. Some budget airlines have restrictions on the type of wheelchair that can be carried. Eurostar trains have two reduced-fare wheelchair areas. There are companies who specialize in travel for those with particular needs; Traveleyes, for example, organize holidays for the visually impaired.

Tourism for All describes itself as the 'UK voice for accessible tourism' and has lots of information for travellers both in the UK and abroad, as well as campaigning for more accessible travel. Enable Holidays can offer a choice of 200 accessible hotels, villas and apartments, all of which have been personally inspected and are graded in their facilities from 'suitable for those with limited mobility' to 'fully wheelchair accessible'. They also offer help with transport. Holidays in specially adapted centres in Essex, Hampshire and Merseyside are run by Vitalise. They offer breaks to travellers with all kinds of disabilities, with or without their carers, and run special holidays for those with Alzheimer's and other dementias. (See Useful addresses for details of all these organizations.)

8

Benefits, finance and practical help

Help is available

Make no mistake about it, there *is* help out there for vulnerable older people, both practical and financial. Money, in the shape of assorted grants and benefits, and disability aids, from wheelchairs and walking frames to mobile phones with especially large and easy-to-use buttons, are all available. All these things are there to make your parents' lives easier, more convenient and more comfortable, and to help them retain their much-cherished independence for as long as it's practically possible. It's understandable that older folk get frustrated and bad-tempered when they can't manage to do the things they want to do, and *need* to do. It makes absolutely no sense for your parents *not* to claim what is rightfully theirs.

Did you know that roughly £5.5 *billion* in pensioners' benefits is left unclaimed each year? Older people often don't claim, for various reasons:

- They are too proud.
- They think that there will be too many complicated forms to fill in.
- They think that benefits are only there for the destitute and because they have some savings or private pensions, or they own their own home, they are not entitled to anything.
- They believe that the amounts involved are so small they're not worth claiming.

Somehow you need to help your parents to understand that these benefits are there for them. They are *entitled* to help from the state after working hard and paying taxes and National Insurance contributions for all those years. That's what it is for! And not all benefits are means tested. Some are available for every older person, regardless of their income or savings.

The 'Social' is there to help them, and people like them. Some old people fear that as soon as Social Services become involved, they will be 'put in a home' regardless of their wishes. In fact, as one hard-pressed social worker said, 'If they only knew . . . we try our very best to support people in their own homes for as long as possible, not only because we know it's what they want but also because it is very much cheaper than taking them into care.'

Yes, there are forms to fill in, but your relatives – and you – can get help with these from organizations like Age UK, Independent Age and the Citizens' Advice. Exactly what an individual will receive in the way of help will depend on their needs, their financial circumstances, and where in the country they live. It also depends on the government of the day. For example, a series of important welfare reforms are due to be introduced, beginning in October 2013. However, these are mostly aimed at people of working age, and according to the government pensioners should receive the same level of help as they do now.

Older people should understand that, *whatever their circumstances*, it is always worth applying for help from the Social Services. If you don't ask, you often don't get – and if you *do* ask, you may be surprised at how helpful the authorities can be.

Here's Norma, aged 91:

> I live alone and although I manage quite well I was nervous about having a bath. I couldn't seem to lift my legs over the side of the bath, and don't have the strength in my arms to pull myself up. I kept thinking how awful it would be if I got stuck and couldn't get out.
>
> My daughter came to stay and told me she thought the Social Services could help. She called them for me and they sent a very nice occupational therapist round about two weeks later. She recommended a bath hoist. I sit on it, push a button, and it lowers me into the bath, and out again when I'm ready! She also arranged for a raised seat for the toilet, with handles at the side so I can get on and off it easily. A couple of weeks later it was all fitted and I didn't have a penny to pay!

Practical equipment like Norma's bath hoist helped with her difficulties. In other circumstances, personal help in the form of paid carers might be the most appropriate way of supporting someone. Or your parent might need both. The way forward is to apply for a *free* community care needs assessment from the Social Services. You can phone your local council Social Services department and ask for this. If your parents' needs are urgent – for example, if they can no longer manage stairs and only have an upstairs bathroom – then say so.

The community care needs assessment

Before this happens, it's a good idea to sit down with your parents and work out exactly what their 'needs' and difficulties are. It's important to let the social worker who comes round get the full picture and understand just what your parents can and can't manage. Don't gloss over anything and make it sound as though your parents can cope when they really can't. If they have good and bad days, describe the worst ones. For example, problems might include:

- getting washed and/or dressed
- cooking meals for themselves
- keeping the house clean and tidy
- climbing stairs
- doing the shopping
- walking – either around the house or outside
- remembering exactly what they have to do and when – whether that means paying the bills or taking their medication on time.

An assessment would normally take place in your parents' home and may involve one or more visits from one or more social workers, or other professionals such as physiotherapists or occupational therapists, depending on the kind of help your parents need.

What your parents will be offered will depend on their level of need and what the particular local Social Services can provide. Help could include the following.

- Carers can provide daily help with washing, dressing, bathing and other personal care.
- A home help might come in to do some housework or even cooking.
- The sort of home adaptations described in Chapter 6 could be carried out: either major items like a stairlift or more minor ones such as grab rails in the bathroom.
- Meals on Wheels can be delivered, or sometimes frozen ready-prepared meals which can be heated in a microwave.

- Assistive technology, or telecare, might be available: items like a pendant, wristlet or even a pressure mat so that a monitoring service, carers or family can be alerted in an emergency.
- A range of respite care and recreation could be on offer: anything from a morning, a day or a couple of days when your parent will be collected, taken to the day centre and brought home again, to a week or so in a care home so that you and your family can have a holiday.

An assessment should take the people's own wishes into account, as well as their physical difficulties, health and housing needs, and whether they have family carers able to provide some care. Social Services should not, however, assume that families are available to provide all the care that is needed. Family carers are entitled to assessments in their own right, too – see Chapter 10.

Once someone has been assessed, the Social Services should provide a 'care plan' detailing exactly what sort of help can be provided. This does vary from place to place. Some councils can help only those whose needs are assessed as 'critical' or 'substantial' rather than 'moderate' or 'low'. If you are not happy with what is offered, you can complain – the Social Services should tell you about their complaints procedure. Get advice from an organization such as Citizens' Advice, or perhaps ask for another assessment later on, when the rules and/or your parents' needs may have changed.

Sometimes, Social Services arrange your parents' care themselves. This can work well, although some people find that they never see the same carers twice, or that carers seem to come at times that suit *them*, rather than the people they are caring for. If this is the case, you can ask whether there could be a way for you or your parents to buy in the services yourselves.

For example, some local authorities offer a Personal Budget arrangement where you are told how much funding is available for you. You are then allowed to take this as a Direct Payment – where you take the cash and arrange and pay for your own care. Or, you may leave the council to commission the services you need, or any combination of the two.

There is also the option of paying for some care privately. If you need, and can afford, to do this, you should contact the UK Homecare Association (see Useful addresses). However, even if this is your choice, make sure you get a care assessment from the Social Services first in case your circumstances change in the future.

Financial help with social care costs

There is no standard system detailing who pays for social care all over the country. It really is a 'postcode lottery' with some councils charging for certain services and not others while others are more generous.

It's best to assume that your parents will have to pay for at least some of the care package they need. This means that it is essential that they claim all the benefits they are entitled to – in other words, their fair share of that £5.5 billion or more that remains unclaimed, as mentioned at the start of this chapter.

The benefits system can seem dauntingly complex, but there is help available from Age UK, the Citizens' Advice, and a very useful website, <www.Turn2us.org.uk>, which has an easy-to-follow online 'benefits calculator'. The idea of the government's welfare reforms is to simplify the system, as well as saving money! The Benefit Enquiry Line on 0800 88 22 00 is another good source of information.

The age at which people can claim their state pension is gradually increasing, and this applies to women born on or after 6 April 1950 and men born on or after 6 April 1953. The Pension Service helpline on 0800 99 1234 can give information about state pension entitlement.

Some additional benefits for older people are not means tested – that is to say, everyone in the appropriate age group gets them regardless of their financial circumstances. The winter fuel payment, designed to help people over 60 with fuel bills, comes into this category, as of course does the bus pass.

Another non-means-tested benefit is the attendance allowance, which is available to anyone over 65 who has 'care needs'. It's paid at two rates – the lower one for those who need 'frequent help or constant supervision during the daytime', and a higher rate for those who need supervision both day and night.

If your parents are on a low income they may be eligible for pension credit, an extremely useful benefit, apparently unclaimed by one in three of those eligible. It is means tested and comes in two parts: 'guarantee credit' tops up a low income to a guaranteed level, and 'savings credit' rewards those over 65 who have modest savings.

It is worth claiming this even if the amount your parents actually get is small, because being in receipt of pension credit entitles them to a whole range of other benefits. For example, their council tax will be paid, they will be entitled to an additional cold weather payment if the temperature drops below a certain level, and they might also be eligible for a warm front grant to insulate their house if needed. The Pension Service can advise on all of this.

If your parents' income is very low they may be eligible for housing benefit (if they rent their home) or council tax benefit. There is also the Social Fund, which gives grants and loans for essential items in particular circumstances to those on low incomes. Again, you can get advice on these from Age UK or the Citizens' Advice.

Any, or all, of these benefit payments can then, of course, be used to pay for extra care around the home, from a home help to clean the house to a regular supply of pre-prepared nourishing meals to stock the freezer.

There are other sources of help, including financial help, for older people on limited incomes. Most professions have 'benevolent funds', which are there to help out people who worked in a particular profession or trade and are struggling to manage in later years. Among the best known are those organizations that support ex-service personnel, such as the Royal British Legion and SSAFA Forces Help (see Useful addresses for contact details). The Turn2us website (see p. 64) has details of many others. Did you know that civil servants, dancers, master mariners and people who worked in the footwear trade are among those who can obtain grants if they are in need? And there are many, many local charitable trusts too, some of whom struggle to give their money away.

It's not all about money

There is no need for your parents' lives to be restricted by old age, frailty, or increasing disability, any more than absolutely necessary. Wheelchairs and other walking aids should be provided by the local NHS, and their GP should be able to refer them to a physiotherapist for an assessment of the kind of equipment that would suit them best and help with using it.

The best source of help in choosing mobility equipment is the fabulous Disabled Living Foundation, based in north-west London, which operates a helpline and an extremely comprehensive website. They produce a full range of factsheets telling you what is available, and there are more than 50 Disabled Living Centres all over the country, where your parents can 'try before they buy'.

It is also worth knowing that you can borrow wheelchairs from the British Red Cross on a short-term basis, which is useful for visitors. Scooters and buggies are not available on the NHS but can be bought or hired. Again, the Disabled Living Foundation is a good source of information. The Shopmobility service lends scooters and wheelchairs free or for a small fee, to allow people with mobility problems easy access to town centres and shopping malls. (See Useful addresses for contact details.)

It's possible that mobility is not the main problem. Perhaps your parents have trouble opening packets and jars, can no longer reach the higher kitchen shelves, struggle to pull on their socks or stockings, find buttons and zips on their clothes fiddly and frustrating, are no longer flexible enough to wash their own hair, or sometimes need to get to the toilet in a hurry. The Disabled Living Foundation can advise on solutions to all these problems.

A wide range of gadgets and gizmos is available to help older and less fit people do everything they need to do. A page on the DLF website, 'Ask Sara', offers custom-made advice. Type in whatever the problem is, then a solution is suggested. Specialist companies such as Hearing and Mobility will send out catalogues of equipment, ranging from 'light touch' pens for people with limited strength in their hands to 'angled measuring jugs' for sufferers from arthritis.

If you know, or suspect, that your relative might be suffering from incontinence, this should be mentioned during the care assessment. It is a problem that their GP should be told about, as it may be the result of an infection. In any case, solutions are available, from laundry services to commodes and specially designed underwear. Get in touch with the Bladder and Bowel Foundation for more help.

Help is also available for those with sight and hearing loss. The telephone is, of course, a priceless lifeline for most older people and today's telephones can be adapted to suit those who are visually impaired or who can't hear very well. You could contact your parents' telephone provider, say that they are old and/or disabled, and ask what concessions they can give. Some companies offer free or reduced rate Directory Enquiries or operator-assisted calls to older customers. They can ask to have their bills sent in Braille or large print.

The Royal National Institute for Blind People has information about the most up-to-date ranges of phones with bigger buttons and spacing, and even talking mobiles!

Similarly, Action on Hearing Loss can tell you about phones with louder ringers or vibrating buzzers, textphones and the Minicom system. They are also the people to contact for information about hearing aids, which are much more sophisticated than they used to be. The T-setting on modern aids allows people to use 'induction loops' so that they can hear more clearly. A loop can be fitted in the home, and public places such as post offices, banks and theatres also have them. Deafness can be extremely isolating, and your parent might need to be reminded to persevere with a new hearing aid which, when used properly, can really transform life! It is also important to remember that other conditions, such as wax build-up, can cause deafness, in which case a hearing aid might not be needed. If one is required your parent will be referred to an audiologist. (For contact details of organizations mentioned, see Useful addresses.)

If money is an issue

Money matters need to be tactfully handled! This is one of those areas – like drinking too much, or incontinence – that it can be terribly difficult to raise with your parents. Some families have never discussed the subject at all and it can be horrifying to find that your elderly dad has been forgetting to pay essential bills or has been taken to the cleaners by a cowboy builder or someone claiming to be from a fraudulent 'lottery'. There are con-men (and women) who prey on the old and vulnerable, and some older people do become forgetful. Others have simply never been very good with money.

The only way to approach this kind of problem is to be open and honest, without being critical, or suggesting that your parent is a silly old fool who has allowed himself to be taken advantage of! No one likes being patronized. In any case, what's done is done, and all you can do is offer help to deal with the situation as you find it.

If your parents have got into debt, the National Debtline (see Useful addresses) is the best source of unbiased advice. Your parents will be helped to prioritize their creditors, first paying something towards essential bills like mortgage or rent and council tax. Harassment by debt collectors is illegal and should be reported to the council's Trading Standards department. Debt advisors can help your parents work out a budget. This is another time to check that they are getting all their benefits.

A more common scenario is when your parents are getting older, and perhaps frailer both physically and mentally, and really can't – or don't want to – deal with all the complexities of savings, bank accounts, investments and bills any longer. Sometimes this happens when the 'half' of the couple who dealt with that side of things dies, and the survivor has never signed a cheque or paid a bill and has no idea where to start.

If your parent is happy for you to take over, that's half the battle. You can obtain a 'third party mandate' from the bank, which your parent signs to allow you access to their bank account. Pensions and benefits are paid directly into bank accounts. People who don't have bank accounts used to be paid by cheque, but this method was phased out from autumn 2012 and replaced by the Simple Payment scheme – a card that is used to collect the money at paypoint outlets in newsagents, supermarkets and other stores. Your parent can arrange for you to collect the money on their behalf by getting you another card. Contact the Department of Work and Pensions on 0800 085 7075 for details of how to do this.

Power of attorney

A 'Lasting Power of Attorney' is a formal arrangement which allows one (or more) people to make important decisions on behalf of someone else. There are currently two types, one concerned with the donor's health and welfare, the other with the donor's property and finances.

In practice, the 'health and welfare' PoA allows someone – yourself – to make decisions about your parent's daily routine and medical care, whether or not they should go into a care home, and what kind of hospital treatment they get. The PoA can only come into force when the donor – your parent – is unable to make their own decisions.

The 'finance and property' PoA allows you to make decisions about things like paying bills, collecting benefits or selling property on behalf of your parent. It can come into force at any time.

The donor must have the mental capacity to agree to the power of attorney being set up and registered with the Office of the Public Guardian (see Useful addresses). There is a fee for this. Forms can be downloaded from the Gov.UK website (<www.gov.uk>) and more information can be obtained from Age UK, the Alzheimer's Society or Citizens' Advice. If your parent has, sadly, lost mental capacity you can apply to the Court of Protection to make decisions for them or to appoint you as a 'deputy' in order to do so.

Clearly, managing someone else's money puts you in a position of trust and you have to act in your parent's best interest at all times. You will need to keep records of their financial circumstances separately from your own.

9

Family matters

If you are an only child, with total responsibility for ageing parents, you can feel tremendously isolated. Everything is down to you. There's no one to help you share decisions, no one to offload your worries on, no one to listen. This is especially true if you are single, of course. However, society is gradually beginning to be aware of just how much care families provide for the old and frail. There are more than 6 million carers in the UK; according to Carers UK, about four out of ten of these are caring for parents or inlaws, and another 16 per cent for other relatives, friends and neighbours. It's estimated that carers save the country £119 *billion* a year. Organizations like Carers Trust (formed by the amalgamation of Crossroads Caring for Carers and the Princess Royal Trust) and Carers UK are working for more and better recognition of the work carers do. You may be an only child, but you are not an only carer, and we shall be looking at the help available for people in your position in Chapter 10.

Having brothers and sisters to share the responsibility, or having a loving partner to help and support you, sounds like a better situation to be in, on the face of it. But as anyone who has found themselves in that position could tell you, it is just not that simple. It's great if you and your siblings get on well, have always done so, and completely agree on the best way to deal with your 'difficult' elders – but what if you don't? A survey in 2011 by Carers UK found that 58 per cent of carers felt that caring had a negative effect on their relationships with other family members, and were worried about this.

Sharing care and sharing major decisions can be an absolute minefield and can lead to anger and resentment on all sides. Someone – usually the sibling who lives nearest to your parents – is relied on most and ends up feeling put-upon. The only sister among a family of brothers can be expected to take on the caring role as a matter of course, simply because she is female. The whole question of inheritance plays a part. Brothers and sisters can suspect each other's motives for suddenly getting in touch with an elderly frail relative, especially if they have never bothered much with Auntie or Gran before. Family circumstances often mean that it's impossible for caring duties to be divided completely equally. If your brother lives in Pakistan or your sister in Australia, he or she can't be expected to fly thousands of miles at a moment's notice.

With goodwill, and good communication on all sides, though, at least some of these issues can be worked out among the family. Problems can be:

- **practical** – in other words, who does what;
- **emotional** – who feels resentful, martyred, 'left-out', unappreciated, guilty;
- **financial** – who pays for what. Families do worry about the 'inheritance' being spent on care.

Practical issues

There are many factors to be considered here. It generally happens that the sibling who lives nearest to the parent is the one who inevitably takes on most of the day-to-day care. Most people are pretty much tied to their current homes by jobs and children's educational requirements, so a house move is not often possible. However, your parents could move – take another look at Chapter 6 for ways in which this can work.

There are other considerations too, of course. What other commitments do you all have? Who is working, full-time or part-time? Who has children, or grandchildren, to care for? Who is in good health? And there are the housing issues we have already seen in earlier chapters. Having an elderly parent move in with you only works if you have space – a spare room, a granny flat, a downstairs bath or shower and toilet, or the possibility of adapting your house to fit these things in. The only way to work it all out is to sit down with your siblings and talk it over. Here's how Julia and her sister Margaret managed when their mother became too frail to live alone.

> I was teaching in a school quite near my home, and my daughter had left home, so I had room for Mum and I had to be there in term-time anyway. I had a cleaning lady whom Mum got on well with in the mornings, and I used Mum's attendance allowance to pay her to stay in the

afternoons until I came home. Mum didn't need nursing, just someone there with her. Mrs D could help her to go to the loo and make a snack lunch for her. In the school holidays, Margaret and her husband – who were retired – came up to stay in my house for part of the time and took Mum back to theirs for a few weeks to give me a break. Mum wasn't the easiest person in the world to care for but Margaret and I agreed that this seemed the best solution. It wouldn't have worked if Margaret and I hadn't got on well, as Mum was very good at playing one of us off against the other!

Emotional issues

As Julia says, you *have* to get on well with your siblings when you are discussing shared care for an older person. Like your relationship with your parents, your relationship with your siblings in the past can affect the way you feel now. It's easy to fall back into the old family roles that you played as children. One of you may still, deep down, feel like the 'big sister' (or brother), the responsible one who automatically took charge when something needed doing. Or, alternatively, you could be the 'family baby' who was always able to twist Mum or Dad round your little finger. One of you could be seen by the others as the 'favoured' child of one parent. Like Julia and Margaret's mother (above), some older people are very good at pushing the buttons and playing on old sibling rivalries.

Can you see how damaging that could be now that you're adults? Big sister feels, 'why is it always me who has to sort things out?' while your other siblings may be either happy to leave it all to you, just as they did when you were children, or else resentful of the fact that once again, you seem to be 'taking over'.

Don't be a control freak who believes that things should be done her – or his – way only. Ask yourself how much it matters if your brother lets Dad stay in his pyjamas all day and drink beer? And be honest about what you want from your brothers and sisters, whether that is practical help or just regular phone calls and a pat on the back!

You can avoid these problems by using family meetings, ideally in person, but otherwise on the phone or via Skype, to sort out relevant issues:

- Talk *and listen* to one another's point of view – including the old folk!

- Share research options that might help (for example, aids to independent living, or carers coming in, or periods of respite care).
- Plan ahead when you can all see that your parents will soon not be able to live alone.
- Think flexibly as circumstances change for your parents, you, and your siblings: for example, your parents may not be able to live with one family member *now*, but that may not always be the case.
- Be absolutely honest with each other about the help you need and are able to give, whether this is practical or financial.

A look at carers' forums on the Internet will show that in some families one sibling is left to get on with the caring, often because the others claim it's 'too upsetting' for them to see or spend time with a seriously ill parent, or one with dementia. 'It's upsetting for me, too,' fumes one carer. 'One of my sisters makes that her excuse, the other tells me I'm doing everything wrong but doesn't offer any helpful suggestions!'

If you're left doing all the work, carers' organizations suggest that you try to find out why your siblings are reluctant to help. Do they, for example, really not know what is needed? Have you told them? They can't be expected to read your mind, especially if they live a long way away and don't see your parents regularly. Are they angry because you seem to have taken over the care without consulting them, and are dealing with everything more competently than they would?

Don't forget, also, that some people are embarrassed or squeamish about anything to do with illness, disability, intimate personal care, or strange behaviour, usually because it is unfamiliar. If your siblings come into that category it can be exasperating. No one likes changing incontinence pads, or explaining to a stranger in a shop or on the bus that Dad doesn't mean to be rude, he has Alzheimer's, but at least you can understand where they're coming from.

If they really can't cope, ask them for the sort of help they *can* give, perhaps doing the shopping or researching paid help or benefits on the Internet.

This is a time to use some real negotiating skills. Tell them how you feel. That doesn't mean accusing them of indifference or selfishness; it means, literally, telling them how you feel – exhausted, worried, or that you're having to do more than your fair share.

If you want them to help, then be specific. Say something like, 'I'd like you to come over for a couple of hours and sit with Mum while I do some shopping', or, 'Could Dad come and stay with you while we have a weekend away/a break/a holiday?'

If they really are not helpful, perhaps someone impartial such as your parents' GP could have a word? There might even be a mediation service in your area where family problems can be discussed. Mediators don't give you the answers, but what they do is bring all parties together and help you to work out a solution, or at least a reasonable compromise.

Sometimes, you just have to accept that the other members of your family simply can't or won't help. Yes, it's sad and unfair, but there comes a point when you are banging your head against a brick wall and achieving exactly nothing. If you're in that position, you need to explore other areas of help and support; for instance, friends, local carers' groups (see Useful addresses) and respite care from the Social Services.

If you are a sibling who really can't offer much practical help – you live too far away, you have a family and/or a very demanding job that you can't afford to give up, or your home is totally unsuitable for a frail old person, make sure the rest of the family knows and understands your situation. Could you help in other ways – possibly financially? Do all the research on benefits so that your parent gets everything they should be claiming? Phone as often as possible and offer a sympathetic, listening ear? The very least you can do is make the carer feel that you appreciate what they're doing rather than taking their hard work for granted.

Financial issues

It's really sad to let the issue of money drive a wedge between you and your nearest and dearest – but it often does. Just because you are siblings, it doesn't mean that you have the same attitudes to money – your own or anyone else's!

If you are handling money on behalf of your parents, either informally or through a power of attorney, it is really vital to keep meticulous records of what you spend and when. Then, if you are ever accused of helping yourself to funds to which you're not entitled, you have proof that this is not so.

If you are making any big financial decisions, such as having Mum or Dad live with you and perhaps using part of the money from the sale of their previous home to pay for an extension to yours, it's best to consult a solicitor and, again, keep careful records of how the money has been spent.

If a parent has to go into care, it's helpful if you and your siblings can agree on which is the most suitable home and how it should be paid for. Some people are reluctant to see their 'inheritance' disappearing into the coffers of an expensive care home – but at the end of the day, it is your parents' money and should be spent for their benefit.

Partners and children

Feeling responsible for elderly parents can become an obsession, to the point where you spend most of your time either caring for them, or worrying that they aren't getting the care they need. It's important to remember that the rest of your family are important too. You can't do everything yourself, and with luck you'll get invaluable support from your partner and children.

It can be stressful for them, too. Their lives, their worries, their concerns, their crises are important and sometimes have to come first. Here's how some carers manage.

> We told Mum well in advance that we were going to help our son and his family move house and that my friend, whom she knew and liked, was going to stay with her while it happened. We kept reminding her, but she still complained a bit and went into her 'no one considers the old folk' routine, but we just tried to ignore her and she was none the worse in the end.

> I found myself as piggy-in-the-middle when Dad first moved in, forever trying to keep the peace between him and his grandsons. In the end it was my husband who told me I should back off as it was worrying me to death. Now, if they 'have words' as they sometimes do, I just think well, that's tough!

Relate (see Useful addresses) offers family counselling, which can be very useful if you feel that your caring responsibilities are driving a wedge between you and your partner and children. Marie is an experienced counsellor:

> Feeling responsible for elderly parents or in-laws is just one of a whole raft of problems couples may encounter. It's a fact of life

but it does get stressful and can really put pressure on, especially if there has always been tension with the in-laws.

It's about priorities. If your mum has always been very demanding and controlling, you may not be able to give enough attention to the rest of your family. If your husband gets fed up, you could both benefit from family counselling to help you see what is really happening. Why are you so dominated by your mother? The question to ask is, how can we face this together and find a way forward? Hopefully you can get your partner on board and he might even tell you you're trying to do too much. You need to realize that the bickering and tension may be caused by the pressure you're under. Even children can understand that you want to do your best for Granny or Granddad but there is only so much you can do.

Stepfamilies

If it's sometimes hard balancing the conflicting demands of elderly parents with those of your partner, children and grandchildren, the picture becomes even more muddled when today's complicated family structures are taken into account. We tend to think that stepfamilies are something new, but of course they're not. It's just that today's stepfamily relationships tend to be the result of divorce, and unofficial, live-in partnerships, whereas in earlier times they were the result of widowhood.

We assume that becoming a stepfamily is only problematic when young children are involved – the 'yours, mine and ours' syndrome. Not much attention is given to the issues that can arise within families when older people marry or form new relationships. And they do. In 2010, according to the Office for National Statistics, more than 4,700 people over 65 remarried. That figure doesn't, of course, include older people in informal partnerships. Not all these later-life relationships are welcomed by the adult children affected, as one stepmother in her sixties put it:

> I don't know why grown-up children can't just be happy for their parents. They don't want to spend all their time with Mum or Dad; they have their own lives to live and would soon be complaining if their parents interfered with that. They should be glad their parent is not alone, has found a loving companion, and is happy!

This is by no means always the case, though, as the following stories show. Adult children seem to be especially upset if a parent remarries 'too soon' after losing their original partner, or if the new partner is a much younger man or woman.

Dad married an old family friend less than two years after Mum died. He sold our family home and seemed to want to get rid of all Mum's things straight away. It was as if he was wiping more than 40 years of marriage out of his life. They moved into her house and spent his money on travelling. When we tried to warn him, gently, that this put him in a very vulnerable position, as her house was willed to her children, it caused a huge family rift.

Dad's new girlfriend was younger than I am, and I couldn't help wondering about her motives, especially when I found out that she had already seen off one very elderly husband!

Mum absolutely hated being on her own and took up with another man she met on the Internet less than six months after my father died. It was a disaster. None of us liked him. Thankfully they didn't marry. The relationship went wrong very quickly and he disappeared from her life. We suspect he had another wife tucked away somewhere!

My father had a heart attack and died just months after he remarried. It put my brother and me in an awful position, having to arrange a funeral and clear Dad's things – and some of Mum's too – alongside a strange woman we had only met a couple of times and hardly knew.

If you are faced with a situation like this, what can you do? First, you have to realize that seeing your parent in a relationship with someone new is always going to feel strange – and, yes, painful. But it doesn't mean that their first partner has been forgotten. In a sense, it's a compliment to them. Your remaining parent is trying to recreate the happiness they had, the first time around. What you have to do is treat the newcomer with the same respect and understanding that you would expect if you brought a new partner home.

The worst thing you can do is assume that Mum or Dad is a silly old fool who is being taken advantage of by some floozie or toy-boy who is after the family silver! We have seen in earlier chapters how much older people dislike being patronized. If you don't feel that you can wholeheartedly welcome the newcomer, at least try to stand back and look at them objectively. You can't help how you *feel* about your parent's new partner, but the least you can do is treat them politely and with friendliness. Give them a chance. It takes time for stepfamilies to 'blend', and a stepfamily is what you now have, even though you might not think of it that way.

There can be advantages to the new arrangement – not least, that you no longer have to worry about a frail elderly parent being alone and lonely. You could find yourself being part of an extended clan if the new partner has family too, and this could mean caring responsibilities can be shared. You may not all get on, but biological families don't always get on either.

Money, the whole issue of inheritance, tends to loom large in families' lists of worries when older people remarry. One of the unintended consequences of the huge rise in house prices in recent years is that even modest family homes in some parts of the UK can now be worth hundreds of thousands of pounds, and legacies can involve life-changing sums of money. You need to be really tactful if you mention this to your parents. Try to make it part of a general discussion about the new living arrangements, rather than making it sound as if your inheritance is all you care about! Christine, quoted above, whose father sadly died very shortly after his remarriage, says:

> Dad had made a point of telling my brother and myself that he and Jean had organized their finances properly when they married. Jean's flat was rented out and she and Dad had bought their house together, so my brother and I were entitled to our share, and were able to buy her out. That was one thing we didn't have to worry about at what was a very fraught time.

10

Taking care of yourself

You might not think of yourself as a 'carer', perhaps because you have an outside job, you don't live with your elderly parents, or the care you give is shared with other family members. However, if you feel responsible for the welfare of your parents, and do your best to take care of them, then you *are* a carer. One of the most vital aspects of caring for someone else – and the one that is most often neglected – is taking care of yourself.

Why self-care is so important

It may seem selfless and devoted to try to do absolutely everything for your elderly parents yourself, but if you step back and think clearly, you'll realize that it is actually very short-sighted. Running yourself into the ground, taking on all the responsibility, without a break, telling yourself and everyone else that of course you can cope, will just exhaust you. Worse, it could end up making you emotionally stressed and possibly physically ill. No one should be expected to 'do it all' – and trying will not help you, the rest of your family, or the parents you care for.

It isn't selfish to remember, as we said right at the beginning of this book, that *you have rights too*. Don't be a martyr, and do take care of yourself. You know it makes sense.

It's important not to get into the sort of mindset that thinks that no one can care for Mum or Dad as well as you can. Strictly speaking, that may be true, and there are some older people who take advantage of your feelings and sulk if you admit to needing a break from caring. But you do. If you're offered informal help – from a sister, brother, friend or neighbour, then take it. If Mum grumbles, let her. There's no need to have an argument, just explain gently that you need a couple of hours to have your hair done/do some shopping/go to the kids' school play or sports day. Sometimes 'granny-sitters' form really close

79

friendships with their 'clients' and you could even end up having your ears bent about what good fun Jenny is or what delicious biscuits she serves.

We looked at the practical and financial help available to frail older people in Chapter 8. If your parent has had a care assessment from the Social Services, some of the help provided will actually benefit you, as the carer, too. For instance, if Dad now has a bath hoist to help him in and out of the bath, that should mean no more lifting for you. If Mum now has a telecare system in place with a button to press if she needs urgent assistance, you won't have so many worries about the fact that she lives on her own and is prone to falls.

Carers' assessments

As well as the care assessment that has to be provided by the Social Services for someone who is old, frail and needing care, you might qualify for a separate carers' assessment, which looks at *your* needs, as a carer, quite separately from those of the person you're caring for.

You are entitled to a carers' assessment if you are providing 'regular' and 'substantial' care for another person, but there is no actual legal definition of this. It's not about the number of hours of caring you provide, although this is, of course, part of it. It all depends on your circumstances – the type of care you give, your other commitments such as a family, and paid work, and the impact of caring on your life. You can apply for one of these assessments if you plan to start caring, even though you haven't yet done so, and whether you actually live with the cared-for person or not.

If you want to investigate this, ask your local Social Services. You will be given an appointment, at which point it's a good idea to contact one of the carers' organizations such as Carers UK. They will help you to prepare for your assessment and tell you what the social worker preparing the assessment will want to know.

Carers UK recommend that you think about the kind of help you would like that would make it easier for you to look after your parent. That's not to say that the Social Services will be able to provide everything you need, but at least it will provide a starting point for discussion. Think about what you actually do for your parent, for example:

- cooking meals for them and doing their shopping
- cleaning their house
- doing their gardening
- collecting their pension and paying bills for them
- personal care, such as getting them up and dressed, helping them to go to the toilet or take a bath.

The social worker will want to know how convenient it is for you to look after your parent. Do you live with them, nearby, or some distance away? How do you travel to their home? Can you drive and do you have access to a car?

What about the health and mobility needs of your parent? Can they walk about without help? Get up from a chair easily? Climb stairs? Have a bath on their own? Are they reasonably fit both physically and mentally? Are there incontinence problems, and if there are how do you deal with them?

How is your own health? For example, if you have a bad back, then lifting your parent might be difficult or even impossible. Do you sleep well? Do you find that your caring responsibilities make you feel stressed, angry, depressed?

It's important that you give the social worker a full picture, rather than claiming that you can cope and understating your difficulties. Tell him or her:

- if your parent needs help at night and how you provide this;
- roughly how many hours a day or week you 'care';
- whether you get any help and how often;
- whether you have a job (or want one) and how understanding your employer is about your situation;
- about your family circumstances and how your other relationships are affected by your being a carer;
- how you feel about the amount of caring you provide – the Social Services should not assume that you can go on providing as much care as you do;
- if you are concerned about what would happen in an emergency – for example, if you had an accident and were taken to hospital. What sort of arrangements could be made for your parent then?

The help you will actually be offered after the assessment will vary, according to your circumstances and where you live, as some Social Services departments are more generous than others. But help might include:

- aids and adaptations such as those described in Chapter 8 to make life easier for you as well as your parent;
- paid carers to help with your parent's personal care;
- Meals on Wheels or similar;
- a laundry service if incontinence is an issue;
- regular breaks from caring for you – either with someone coming in to care for your parent or them being offered respite care in a day centre or care home;
- useful information about benefits, counselling, or local carers' groups you can join.

In some areas Social Services provide this sort of help directly. In others it is provided by voluntary organizations or private companies. Or you could receive Direct Payments, which allow you to buy in the recommended care yourself. (See Chapter 8 for more on Personal Budget/ Direct Payments.) The advantage of this is that you (and your parent) can choose exactly what you need and make arrangements that suit you all. Direct Payments are completely flexible and you could, for instance, use them to pay for driving lessons, stress management classes, or even a short holiday.

It varies between areas as to whether different care services are free or have to be paid for, but charges have to be 'reasonable'. If you are not happy with your assessment, the services provided, or the charges made for them, it's a good idea to contact one of the carers' organizations who can help you with the complaints procedure.

Other support for carers

Carers' groups

Looking after your elderly parents can sometimes make you feel very isolated, which is why so many carers' groups have been set up. You can find out about groups available locally by contacting your GP, Carers UK or the Carers Trust. Some groups are for all carers, others are specifically for those caring for older people or those with Alzheimer's or other dementias. They are usually run by and for the members and can be a lifeline for those who need to share information, have a break, have a laugh or find a shoulder to cry on! Here's Linda on her local carers' group.

> I was desperate, when I saw the group advertised in my GP's surgery and it proved to be a lifeline. I have made so many friends and they are all people who know just what I'm going through with Mum because they have been through the same themselves. I think what I needed more than anything else was someone to listen. We organize weekend breaks and days out and I feel as though I've been given my life back. I have also had all sorts of tips on the best way to deal with Mum and some help with claiming benefits too, all from people who had experience of the same problem. I don't know what I would have done without the group, they have absolutely changed my life.

The medical profession

Make sure that you tell your GP that you are a carer. Some practices offer special carers' services such as health checks, or early morning and late evening appointments to fit in with your responsibilities.

If your parent has to go into hospital, the hospital should give you a named contact on the ward so that you know whom to call if you need to. You should, of course, be involved in your parent's care while they are in hospital and also after they come out, when they might need extra help from a community nurse, social worker or therapist.

Carer's allowance

You can claim this not-very-generous benefit – currently £58.45 per week – for yourself if you 'care' for 35 hours a week or more, and, if you're working, you earn less than £100 a week. However, you will not be entitled to it if you are already receiving some other benefits. If you are receiving a state pension of more than a certain amount, you won't be eligible for the carer's allowance but you may be eligible for a 'carer premium', which could reduce your council tax bill or increase your other benefits. Confusing? Yes, it can be, so call the Carers UK advice line for help in your particular circumstances.

Dealing with feelings

It's important to get all the practical help you can when you have elderly parents to look after, but looking after them isn't just about grab rails and day centres. Feelings matter too. One of the advantages of belonging to a carers' group is that you'll learn that other people in the same situation have the same feelings as you do.

What might those feelings be? Sadness, because you are watching your parents get older, frailer and less capable. Anger, resentment and exasperation will be part of the package too. You're not a saint and caring for someone who is slow, contrary or just plain bloody-minded can try your patience to the limit. There will also be guilt, because whatever you do seems to be wrong, or not enough, and you may be continually criticized and found fault with.

You'll need to acknowledge and accept your feelings, but at the same time accept that you are doing your best, and no one can do more. If your parents are difficult and critical you need to remind yourself, as we found in earlier chapters, that a lot of their frustration isn't really directed at you, but at the situation they are in. You can make sure they are warm, well fed, comfortable, and have all the help that can be provided to make their lives easier and more pleasant – but you can't make them young again. You can't make them happy. You can't bring back the old friends they have lost. The world has moved on, and if the world of tablet computers and MP3 players is frustrating and confusing for them, it's no one's fault.

Consultant clinical psychologist Dr Pat Frankish says:

> Feeling guilty is something everyone is capable of and anyone with emotionally blackmailing parents will have grown up feeling guilty. Depression is linked with feelings of guilt. If your parents make you feel guilty, you will not be alone. Attending a carers' group will help you to find a peer group with the same issues. The bottom line is, we can only do our best, and that best depends on our personal internal resources. The better the parenting experienced, the more personal resources are available. It follows that parents who do a good job will be more likely to have adult children who want to help them.

Marie, an experienced Relate counsellor, points out that adult children often make excuses for their parents' bad behaviour and that it can help to acknowledge that your Mum is badly behaved!

Think carefully about the commitments you make. Having a row does not help but you can negotiate and change the balance a bit by being assertive and saying something like 'I wish I could help, but tomorrow I have to . . . could I come round on Friday instead?' You may need to be determined and confident and stick to your guns.

Take time out for yourself

Looking after yourself is a vital part of being a carer. It's not selfish or self-indulgent, it's essential. Eating a healthy, balanced diet, sleeping well, including some exercise in your daily routine, learning to relax and enjoy 'me' time that takes you right away from your caring role, will all make you a better carer.

It may seem like a tall order, if you are juggling a home, family and a job with responsibility for your parents, but none of the elements of healthy living mentioned above need take up hours of time. Preparing a healthy meal – say, a grilled chop with potatoes and vegetables, or a baked jacket potato with a cheese or tuna-and-sweetcorn filling plus salad – doesn't take any longer than a less healthy meal.

In fact, healthy eating can be easier than you think. Avoid full-fat dairy products – go for semi-skimmed milk and low-fat cheese. Buy wholemeal bread and pasta and brown rice. Save very sweet, stodgy or creamy puddings for special occasions and serve fruit after meals instead.

Busy, stressed people often find it hard to wind down, relax and sleep properly. Are you one of those who can't 'switch off' at night, whose mind continues to race even after you've gone to bed, thinking about the events of the day and fretting about everything you have to do tomorrow? If that's you, you are certainly not alone! You might benefit from one of the 'relaxation therapies' mentioned below, such as yoga, t'ai chi or autogenic training. Or try some simple tips:

- Develop a soothing bedtime routine – a warm bath with a relaxing oil such as lavender, followed by a milky drink and some undemanding TV or a book.
- Leave several hours between your evening meal and going to bed. People don't sleep well if they have indigestion!
- Don't be tempted to have an alcoholic nightcap. Alcohol may seem to help you get off to sleep but it often wakes you in the small hours, which is not what you need. It is also a depressant.

- Pay attention to 'sleep hygiene'. Make sure your bedroom is quiet and comfortable, not too hot or chilly, and keep work and TV out of the bedroom. Beds are for sleeping in!
- Get to know your body clock. If you're a natural lark, who finds it easy to get up in the morning but droops after about 10 p.m., make the most of it. The same applies if you're an owl who isn't really sleepy until after midnight.
- Try not to worry if you have the odd bad night. You probably sleep more than you think you do. Tell yourself you are warm and safe in bed and let tomorrow's worries take care of themselves. Let yourself daydream . . . you're on a sunlit holiday beach or curled up before a roaring fire . . . and you'll soon drop off.
- If lack of sleep leaves you feeling totally drained and exhausted, go to your GP.

Finding time to exercise can also sound like a daunting prospect when you're busy, but it doesn't have to be. You don't have to join a gym or take up running – though if either of those appeals, then why not? It's often simpler to incorporate some exercise into your everyday routine. Walk to work or the shops, or at least catch the bus a few stops further on. Walk up the stairs instead of using the lift. Do a few bending and stretching exercises while you're waiting for the kettle to boil or the microwave to 'ping'.

As well as being good for your physical health, exercise is very good at lifting mild depression and taking you away from your everyday worries. You might think you're not the sporty type but there must be something active that you'd enjoy doing – alone, with a friend, or with the rest of the family. Walking, dancing, swimming, Pilates, cycling – why not pop into your local leisure centre and see what's on offer?

How often are you able to relax, *really* relax? In today's fast-paced world we spend our lives rushing from one commitment or activity to the next. Modern communications mean that we are expected to be 'on duty' 24/7, checking our emails on the train and answering our mobiles wherever we are. No wonder we get stressed.

The only way to deal with this is to STOP. Somehow, we all have to convince ourselves that it's OK – in fact it's more than OK, it's vital – to spend some time doing absolutely nothing. If you find it hard to switch off, and feel that when you try to your mind is still racing, consider taking up some sort of relaxation therapy. Your GP may be able to suggest local stress management classes, or you could contact the governing bodies for activities such as yoga, t'ai chi, meditation or autogenic training (see Useful addresses). All these therapies are intended to help you slow down, switch off and refresh both body and mind.

Or you could take up a truly absorbing hobby – anything from tracing your family tree to collecting antique jewellery or 1930s china. Men tend to be better at this than women, hence the number of 'golf widows'! They have a point, though. Even an hour doing something you enjoy, something completely different, can help you to see your everyday worries in perspective.

11

When you've done your best

What happens, though, when you've done all you can, and it still isn't good enough? We have seen throughout this book that there is a lot of help available for frail older people, both financial and practical. There are also tactful ways that worried families and friends can suggest that they accept the help they are offered. Suggest, though, is the operative word. The hard fact is that no one can actually *make* an older person – or anyone else for that matter – accept help if they are unwilling to do so.

It's a problem that social workers and health professionals come up against all the time. I asked an experienced social worker how his team dealt with people who were difficult to help.

People who absolutely refuse to have *anything* to do with *anyone* are actually quite rare. One useful thing to remember is that the time may not be right, at this moment, to intervene. It may not even be necessary for help to be accepted right now, but if you mention or suggest something, sow the seed as it were, in time you might find the person changes their mind. No one likes being told what to do, so it's better not to go in with all guns blazing. If you have regard for their dignity and self-respect and suggest some help, they might end up by thinking it was all their own idea in the first place.

Families sometimes need to be a bit devious. For example, you might suggest a home carer or volunteer or even a neighbour who could do a bit of shopping for your parents. Then, when a relationship has been established, that could be the time to suggest the person helps with the cleaning or cooking or gardening as well.

If they won't be helped at all, if they have chosen not to be, then they do have the right to refuse intervention. That might be worrying for their families, who may have to accept that they can't solve everything or take away all risk from their parents' lives. It can help to talk it over with a professional, who can advise them if they are worrying unnecessarily, or fellow carers.

It's important to take the person's mental capacity into account. Not all old people have reduced mental capacity, but many do. Some may lack insight into their own capacity. They may, for example, be convinced that they have cooked themselves a meal, or put the heating on, when they haven't. The Mental Capacity Act 2007 – an amendment to the Mental Health Act 2005 – is there to deal with situations where people are no longer able to make safe decisions for themselves. However, the tests for mental capacity are quite high and if someone says, 'I'm not going into a home!' they may very well be assessed as having the capacity to make that decision.

Generally, social workers will consider invoking the Mental Health Act only when there is a more extreme situation. Perhaps the person is seriously neglecting himself, or is violent, and/or at significant risk. Then an intervention by a mental health team might be needed. Families are often reluctant to consider this but the psychiatric and social services are there to help. It's often worth looking at your local authority website to see what services are available. Organizations like Age UK and carers' groups are also useful. But there are no easy answers.

What if the problem is, in a sense, the opposite one? It's not that your parent won't accept help, it's that he or she thinks that you, and you alone, should be the person to provide it? After all, you are their son or daughter, they brought you up, so you 'owe' them care in their old age. If you don't provide it, or the amount of care you provide doesn't come up to their exacting standards, woe betide you.

It's a tough question, isn't it? Just how much do you owe your parents? We said in Chapter 1 that they have rights, but so do you. Balancing those rights, when your parents are old and frail and need help, can never be easy. There are cultures where respect and care for older members of the family, *within* the family, are taken for granted and the idea of finding residential care for Gran or Granddad is simply never considered. However, it is worth pointing out that this is more common in societies where fewer women work outside the home, and where life expectancy is lower than it is in the UK, so that there are fewer very old, very frail people to be cared for.

Most people feel that they *should* care for older family members, but as we have seen, there are all sorts of reasons why this might not be appropriate in every case – unsuitable housing, lack of facilities for older people in the area, extreme frailty, which means your parent needs professional nursing care, financial considerations, your commitment to other members of the family. What happens when your love for, and loyalty to, your parents conflicts with your love for your partner, or your children? They deserve consideration too. Guilt, however, seems to come as part of the package, whatever you do.

Carol, whose mother died suddenly – and alone – seven years ago, has this to say:

> I still feel I let Mum down. Our relationship was never easy. She was very affectionate and loving but, in a sense, that was the problem. Like many women of her generation she had never been able to fulfil her potential, but had to leave school and help support the family. She looked to me to fulfil all her ambitions, and when I didn't, I don't think she ever forgave me. I worked 200 miles away and she complained constantly that I didn't visit often enough. When I did visit, she monopolized my time, refusing to welcome my friends to the house or allow me to go out and see them. I phoned her twice a day, morning and evening, and invited her to come and live with me at one point, but she refused to leave Newcastle.
>
> Gradually I became aware that her memory was going. A neighbour told me that he had found her eating raw fish fingers because she had forgotten to cook them. She became confused in the shops and stockpiled vegetables, which all went rotten. But she completely rejected the idea of Meals on Wheels or any help in the house. I'd gladly have paid for central heating and a new kitchen but she wouldn't hear of it. Her GP asked her if she had thought of moving to a care home, and a few days later she was found dead in her bed. A policewoman attended and said, 'How could her family have let her live in such a squalid house?', which hurt me terribly because I had tried, I really had. The guilt just never goes away.

So much depends on the quality of the relationship you have – and always have had – with your parent. People can't help getting old, but they *can* help being critical, demanding, abusive, bullying and downright cantankerous! Living in a three-generation family, as we've seen, is not always easy. It demands compromise – on *both* sides. Older people can't be allowed to become domestic tyrants, making the whole family miserable.

'This is something that we don't discuss very much in our society,' says the social worker. 'Just because people are old and need help, it doesn't change the family history, which may be one of abuse. Not all families get on and the idea that every old person is a dear old lady or gentleman is highly misleading!'

What can you do if your relationship with your parents has always been dysfunctional? Just as not everyone is cut out to be a carer, not everyone is a model parent, or even an adequate one. How much do you owe your parents if you have been bullied or abused or emotionally blackmailed for most of your life? Consultant clinical psychologist Dr Pamela Frankish says:

The temptation in this situation is to go for revenge, to make the parents pay for past sins. Clearly, this is not appropriate if the older person is frail and vulnerable – but it is understandable to have these feelings. If they are too strong for contact to be safe, then adult children should restrict themselves to working with care professionals to make sure that everything practical has been done to help, including home adaptations and support if it's needed.

Unfortunately, people who have had parents who have not provided enough nurture will find it difficult to care, as they will be emotionally stunted by their own experience. Dealing with the guilt may require counselling help.

There is no reason to feel guilty about not providing for someone who did not provide for you. There is reason to feel guilty if you actively harm your parent after they have become vulnerable.

If you had an abusive or neglectful parent, you do not owe them more than they gave you. If you choose to help them, then be aware of why you are doing it. If you feel better, then carry on. If you feel resentful, then stop. And if your elderly parent is still bullying you, or intruding on your sense of self, or ruining your relationship with your partner and children, then you need to protect yourself from them.

It is OK to give up on your parents if they have not been able to give you the start in life that would leave you wanting to be with them and happy to help them.

In the summer of 2012, *The Guardian* newspaper published the story of a woman who had cut off all contact with her parents, as had two of her three siblings, saying that the relationship had completely broken down. Her mother was not old, frail and demanding, but she was a complete narcissist and had always been emotionally abusive.

> She exhausted me, drained me. I got nothing from her because she gave nothing. I was depressed, ill, ground down. I had to get out. Since the break, my depression has lifted. I've lost weight, I carry myself more confidently and I've made changes that have put my life on a much better track. Most importantly, I know I'm not the fatally flawed, bad person my parents used to make me think I was.

She now runs a website, <www.daughtersofnarcissisticmothers.com>, to offer support to those who, like herself, feel that the relationship has completely broken down and is causing nothing but harm.

Of course, it is terribly sad when a family relationship is so toxic, and probably few people would have the courage to make a complete break with their parents. If this is the road you choose, you will certainly benefit from some kind of counselling or therapy, even if it's only to deal with the inevitable questions from friends and acquaintances.

You might also like to consider getting in touch with an organization called NAPAC – the National Association for People Abused in Childhood (see Useful addresses). They will offer a listening ear to anyone who has been physically, emotionally or sexually abused by a parent, or any other adult. Bullying, neglect and a lack of love and care can be every bit as damaging as physical abuse. According to spokesperson Peter Saunders:

> We spend our time listening. Callers are free to offload painful memories to our brilliant team of volunteers. We are not there to judge and it's OK if they express anger or hatred towards the parents who abused them. Many of our callers are middle-aged or elderly and some have never spoken about what happened to them, even to their partners.
>
> We do hear from people who have cared for abusive parents in later life, which is always very challenging. The fact that there was abuse is a huge burden to bear as both parent and child get older. Some still feel that they should 'do their duty' by their parent; others are able to abandon them and admit that they are glad and relieved when the parent dies. Parents have huge power. They

know their children love them in spite of everything and some take advantage of that. It is hard to 'honour' a father who raped you, or a mother who is bitter and angry and refuses to cooperate with those trying to care for her. Some of our callers feel guilt, or regret that their parent wasn't more charitable. Others, including some older people whose parents are long dead, just want to talk to someone and to be able to move on.

Bereavement

Losing someone you love always throws up a range of emotions and this is especially so if you have been a 'carer' – either formally or informally, full-time or part-time. If you have spent years caring for your parent, you are losing your role when you lose them, and this can be difficult in itself. Guilt, as we have seen, is often part of the reaction. Some carers are tormented by the idea that they didn't do enough, see Mum or Dad often enough, or left things unsaid and problems unresolved, and now it's too late.

You'll need to remind yourself that there is no right way to grieve, and this is especially true if you had a fraught relationship with the person who has died. Don't be too hard on yourself. You did what you could. Be your own best friend and don't beat yourself up for all the things you didn't do – think of what you *did* do instead. When you are grieving it's easy to forget just how awkward your parent could be. Try to remember them as they really were – a flawed human being, just like the rest of us.

Ritual can help. The Chinese believe that smoke from incense carries thoughts and wishes straight to heaven. Write your parent a note, saying all the things you wish you had been able to say, and then burn it.

Paul Williams, from the charity Cruse Bereavement Care, says that the Cruse helpline (see Useful addresses) offers people who have been bereaved in any circumstances a safe and non-judgemental space to talk about how they feel.

Our viewpoint is that *every* bereavement is unique to that relationship. Those who call us are often both physically and mentally exhausted, having put all their energy and effort into caring. We can help them to access any support they need and show them how they can look after themselves. Inertia can be a problem but bereaved people do need to eat and sleep and do some exercise.

Sometimes they remember the better parts of the relationship, telling themselves that perhaps Mum was only demanding because she was ill. It's important not to ignore the less good memories, but time may help you to put them into context. Emotions can be very mixed at first and may change with time. Everyone has to find their own way of coping but we are always here. They can talk to us, or write a letter saying everything they would have liked to say to their parent.

Friends can help just by being there and available for the bereaved person. Instead of simply telling them they can always call you, a friend could take the initiative and call the bereaved person. It's important to be sensitive to where the bereaved person is – do they want to be distracted, or just someone to listen? Sometimes 'I'm so sorry' is all you can say.

Useful addresses

Abbeyfield
Tel.: 01727 857536; www.abbeyfield.com
Supported housing for older people.

Action for Advocacy
Tel.: 020 7921 4395; www.actionforadvocacy.org.uk

Action on Hearing Loss
Helpline: 0808 808 0123; www.actiononhearingloss.org.uk

Admiral Nurses
Helpline: 0845 257 9406; www.dementia.uk.org
Help and advice from trained dementia care nurses.

Age UK
Helpline: 0800 169 6565; www.ageuk.org.uk

Al-Anon
Tel.: 020 7403 0888; www.al-anonuk.org.uk
Help for the friends and families of problem drinkers.

Alcoholics Anonymous
Helpline: 0845 769 7555; www.alcoholics-anonymous.org.uk

Alzheimer's Society
Helpline: 0300 222 1122; www.alzheimers.org.uk

Anxiety Care UK
Tel: 07552 877219; www.anxietycare.org.uk

Asperger's Syndrome Foundation
C/o Littlestone Golding
Eden House
Reynolds Road
Beaconsfield HP9 2FL
www.aspergerfoundation.org.uk

Benefit Enquiry Line
Tel.: 0800 882200; www.gov.uk/benefit-enquiry-line

Bipolar UK
Tel.: 020 7931 6480; www.bipolaruk.org.uk

Bladder and Bowel Foundation
Helpline: 0845 345 0165; www.bladderandbowelfoundation.org

British Association for Counselling and Psychotherapy
Tel.: 01455 883300; www.bacp.co.uk

British Autogenic Society
Tel.: 07534 539425; www.autogenic-therapy.org.uk

British Red Cross
Helpline: 0844 412 2804; www.redcross.org.uk
Short-term support for vulnerable people, including loan of equipment.

British Wheel of Yoga
Tel.: 01529 306851; www.bwy.org.uk

Carers Trust
Helpline: 0844 800 4361; wwws.carers.org

Carers UK
Advice line: 0808 808 7777 (Wednesdays and Thursdays, 10 a.m. to
12 noon/2 p.m to 4 p.m.); www.carersuk.org

Cinnamon Trust
Tel.: 01736 757900; www.cinnamon.org.uk
For bereaved pet-owners and their pets.

Citizens' Advice
For phone contact details, please refer to a directory for details of your
local branch of Citizens' Advice.
www.citizensadvice.org.uk

Contact the Elderly
Helpline: 0800 716 543; www.contact-the-elderly.org.uk
Befriending service for isolated older people.

Cruse Bereavement Care
Helpline: 0844 477 9400; www.cruse.org.uk

Department for Work and Pensions
Tel.: 0800 885 7075; www.gov.uk/dwp

Depression UK
C/o Self Help Nottingham
Ormiston House
32–36 Pelham Street
Nottingham NG1 2EG
www.depressionuk.org

Disability Rights UK
Tel.: 020 7250 3222; www.disabilityrightsuk.org

Disabled Living Foundation
Helpline: 0845 130 9177 (10 a.m. to 4 p.m., weekdays); www.dlf.org.uk

Drink Aware
Tel.: 020 7766 9900; www.drinkaware.co.uk
For information on the effects of alcohol.

Elderly Accommodation Counsel
Helpline: 0800 377 7070; www.eac.org.uk
Information on housing options for older people.

Enable Holidays
Tel.: 0871 222 4939; www.enableholidays.com
Information on holidays for people with disabilities.

Forum of Mobility Centres
Helpline: 0800 559 3636; www.mobility-centres.org.uk
Information for disabled drivers and passengers.

Hearing and Mobility
Helpline: 0844 888 1338; www.hearingandmobility.co.uk
Runs stores and online shopping for disability aids.

Independent Age
Advice line: 0845 262 1863 (10 a.m. to 4 p.m., Monday to Friday); www.
independentage.org
Advice and support for older people.

Macmillan Cancer Support
Helpline: 0808 808 0000; www.macmillan.org.uk

MIND
Infoline: 0300 123 3393; www.mind.org.uk
For help with all mental-health issues.

NAPAC
Support line: 0800 085 3330; www.napac.org.uk
Support for people abused in childhood.

National Debtline
Helpline: 0808 808 4000; www.nationaldebtline.co.uk

National Institute of Medical Herbalists
Tel.: 01392 426022; www.nimh.org.uk

National Trust
Tel.: 0844 800 1895; www.nationaltrust.org.uk

No Panic
Helpline: 0800 138 8889; www.nopanic.org.uk
For help with phobias and panic attacks

Office of the Public Guardian
Helpline: 0300 456 0300; www.justice.gov.uk/about/opg
Information about Powers of Attorney.

Older People's Advocacy Alliance
Tel.: 01782 844036 (administrator); www.opaal.org.uk

Pension Service
Helpline: 0800 99 1234; www.gov.uk/contact-pension-service

Pets as Therapy
14a High Street
Wendover
Aylesbury HP22 6EA
www.petsastherapy.org

Relate
Helpline: 0300 100 1234; www.relate.org.uk
Help with all relationship issues.

Rethink
Helpline: 0300 5000 927; www.rethink.org
For information on all kinds of mental illness.

Retired and Senior Volunteer Programme
Tel.: 020 7643 1385; www.csv-rsvp.org.uk

RNIB
Helpline: 0303 123 9999; www.rnib.org.uk
Help for blind and partially sighted people.

Royal British Legion
Helpline: 08457 725 725; www.britishlegion.org.uk
Help and support for those who have served in the Forces and their families.

Royal Voluntary Service (formerly Women's Royal Voluntary Service (WRVS))
Helpline: 0845 600 5885; www.royalvoluntaryservice.org.uk
Personal and practical support for older people.

St John Ambulance
Tel.: 020 7324 4000; www.sja.org.uk

Salvation Army
Tel.: 020 7367 4500; www.salvationarmy.org.uk
Practical support and help for older people.

Samaritans
Helpline: 08457 90 90 90; www.samaritans.org
Support line for anyone: available 24 hours a day, 7 days a week.

Shopmobility
Helpline: 0844 4141 850; www.shopmobilityuk.org
Loans wheelchairs and mobility scooters.

SSAFA Forces Help
Tel.: 020 7403 8783; www.ssafa.org.uk
Help for serving and former service personnel and their families.

Tourism for All
Helpline: 0845 124 9971; www.tourismforall.org.uk

Traveleyes
Helpline: 0844 804 0221; www.traveleyes-international.com
Help for visually impaired travellers.

UK Homecare Association
Helpline: 020 8661 8188; www.ukhca.co.uk
Information on companies providing paid-for care in the home.

University of the Third Age
Tel.: 020 8466 6139; www.u3a.org.uk

Vitalise
Helpline: 0303 303 0145; www.vitalise.org.uk
Holidays for people with disabilities, including dementia.

Index